# THE ULTIMATE

## TREATMENT COORDINATOR

### Closing Secrets of the Nation's Top 1% Orthodontic Practices

**Luke Infinger**

# The Ultimate Treatment Coordinator

ISBN-13: 978-1-990476-06-8

Published by: Expert Author Press

https://www.expertauthorpress.com/

Canadian Address:

1908 – 1251 Cardero Street,

Vancouver, BC, Canada, V6G 2H9

Phone: (604) 941-3041

info@expertauthorpress.com

# Table of Contents

# Acknowledgements

A big thank you to Kasey Workman, Vanessa Fitzwater, Mary Scott, Madison Martin, and Stacey Bagwell, the wonderful Treatment Coordinators who contributed their time, knowledge, and insights about the TC role into this book; as well as Beverly Simkins, Lead Scheduling Coordinator, for showing us how collaboration and teamwork between scheduling coordinators and treatment coordinators keeps the office running like a well-oiled machine.

To Dr. Ben Fishbein, the owner of the legendary Fishbein Orthodontics, thank you for being an exemplary leader and innovator; we are humbled by your dedication to your team, patients, and the orthodontic profession. To Knecht Orthodontics, thank you for allowing us to showcase your growth journey in this book. To Dr. Keith Dressler, thank you for being a great friend and mentor. And to Harrison Bagdan, the Senior Practice Advisor at HIP, your contributions to this book are very much appreciated.

A final thank you to everyone who made this book possible!

# A Note from the Author

The economy is always changing and whatever the direction of the flux, there are some people who are scared, others who are anxious, and some who eagerly embrace whatever is coming their way. As I write these words, it's the end of the second quarter of 2022, and the world has moved from one state of turmoil to another. The experts are talking about a recession and warn that tough times are ahead.

I don't know about you, but I've heard these doom and gloom predictions many times in my life, and sure, what we could count on one day was not always the same the next. However, there are always people doing great things, building amazing businesses, and changing lives, regardless of the economics of the day. I want you to be one of them.

Here's the thing. Attitude is everything. Those people who seem to thrive no matter what's going down around them have a mindset of success that is clear to everyone. You might think I'm trying to give you a pep talk, and maybe I am, but my purpose is twofold. As an orthodontist or a leader in an orthodontic practice, it's your duty to inspire people to take care of their number one attitude-enhancing asset. That's right, I'm talking about the gorgeous smiles you help people create. Therefore, your winning attitude helps people decide to start treatment and build the smile they need to inspire others.

It's a tall order, but in any economy, here are some stats on the smile:

- 80% of adults report that straightening their teeth was one of the most important treatments of their lives.
- 76% admit that a smile is the #1 physical trait to make a first impression.

- According to 68% of Americans, people who smile are more trustworthy, confident, and approachable.

My point is that you signed up for this. It's your job to keep the world smiling and in order to do that, you have to help influence new patients to start care at your practice. In fact, I think your responsibility is so vast that this entire book is dedicated to the strategies you need to get new patients to start treatment. You'll even learn how some of the top 1% orthodontic practices in the nation are getting people to start on the same day they do their complimentary consultation.

I hope you have fun with this and get your entire team on board so that together, you can help your community thrive.


Best,

**Luke Infinger**
Co-Founder & CEO at HIP

# About Luke

"If I hire you, will you stop bugging me?" asked the manager at Chick-fil-A with a resigned, yet slightly amused look. I had shown up, resume in hand, asking to speak to him every week for the past three months. Until that day, every week he had said, "No, you're too young." I was 15 years old at the time.

He must have realized that my persistence and dedication were useful traits in an employee, and they were. Chick-fil-A's customer service values became my own, and soon I was put in charge of delivering packets with motivational training from Zig Ziglar and Jim Rohn to all new employees. I learned that if you believe in yourself and whatever you're selling, persistence pays off.

My next two jobs were commission sales jobs. One was with Buckle, a retail chain with stores located in malls, and the other was selling the New York Times by phone. In both jobs, I became one of the top salespeople. I quickly learned that if you know all the ins and outs of your product, and believe in it, you can transfer that belief and gain trust.

I went on to study motion graphics at the Savannah College of Art & Design (SCAD). When I graduated, I targeted a motion graphics shop in New York City and sent LinkedIn messages to every single person until a former SCAD graduate got me in for an interview. The hours were awful and the culture was worse, but for the year I was there, I crushed it. I did the entire third season promos for Game of Thrones with the help of one other guy.

I left there and started HIP. My early career path taught me that training in personal growth, customer service, and sales creates magic in teams. A positive and supportive culture is paramount. If you take an interest in your employees and are caring, yet firm, they will show up excited and eager to serve.

At HIP, we know everything about the business of orthodontics, not just marketing. We are invested in the vision that you have for your life, your team, and your community. That's why we partner with the practices we serve.

My mission is to live with integrity and help business owners make the best decisions with their time, money, marketing, and health. I repeat this to myself daily as part of my morning formula to make sure it is reflected in all aspects of my life. Life is about more than just work. That's why I care about WHY our partners want to grow their business and the lifestyle they want to create.

When I'm not working, I enjoy spending time with my wife Kathryn and our daughter Aislinn Rhys, who's 4, going on 5. You'll find me in the garden, reading books or studying health and natural living.

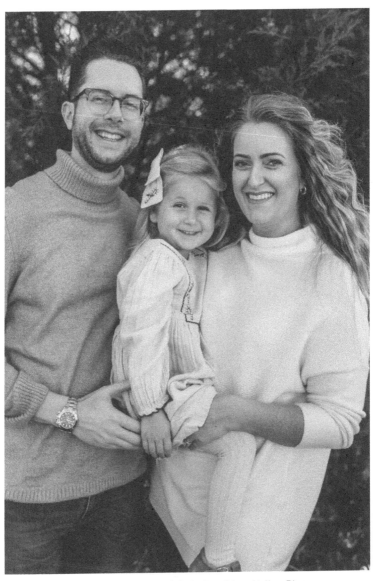

*Luke, Kathryn, and their daughter, Aislinn Rhys*

# Introduction

New patients are the lifeblood of every orthodontic practice. Without a fresh batch of starts each month, every practice would shrink to nothing in a couple of years. That's why the number one comment I hear from orthodontists, and I talk to hundreds every year, is, "I just need more new patients."

Because my company, HIP, specializes in orthodontic practice growth and marketing, the conversation quickly moves to, "Can YOU get us more new patients?" We start to talk about websites and running ads to generate leads and pretty soon they're telling me that, "Leads from the internet are low quality."

One guy asked if we could block "certain types" of people from seeing his ads and website.

Another asked, "Can we rank the leads? Maybe give them a grade like A, B, C, and D? Because I only want to follow up with As and Bs."

This one orthodontist who signed on with us said, "Take the request a free consultation form off my website. If they really want to come see us, they can call us. Website leads are ALL BAD patients."

Now, I've worked with hundreds of orthodontic practices since 2014. I've helped some of the nation's fastest-growing orthodontic practices add millions of dollars to their production. Dr. Ben Fishbein has been a client of HIP since our inception and we have helped him grow from 3 locations, 25 staff, and 2 million in production to 8 locations, 100+ staff, and over 25 million in production. Many of our strategies have been tried, tested, and refined in his office.

The one thing I can tell you about growing a practice through online leads is,

*"There are no bad leads."*

This is Book #2 in *The Orthodontic Practice Growth Series.* Book #1, Front Desk Secrets of the Nation's Fastest Growing Orthodontic Practices, is all about how your scheduling coordinator can book more of those leads for free consultations by following one simple principle: Speed to Lead. Throughout this book, as we refer back to Book #1, we

will call it, *Front Desk Secrets*. If you have not read it, please get a few copies and review it with your team. You can order them here, or reach out to me and I'll gladly send some to your office.

The principles, processes, and scripts in that book alone can easily add hundreds of thousands of dollars to production. More importantly, you'll see firsthand how offices just like yours are turning "low quality online leads" into new patient consultations and starts.

Our focus in Book #2 is on the Treatment Coordinator (TC) role. Your TC is the person responsible for inspiring the new patients to make the commitment to the process of straightening their teeth and building a winning smile. After the new patient has had their consultation and the doctor has given their recommendations for treatment, we want them to say 'yes' to the process and make financial arrangements to pay the $5000-$7000 cost. We refer to this as the conversion of a new patient consultation to a start. The national average for conversion in orthodontic offices is 52% or roughly one out of every two new patients agreeing to follow the recommendations and begin paying.

How does your clinic stack up to the national average? If you're at or slightly above average, maybe you're feeling pretty good about yourself and your team, and you should. However, life is about growth and evolution, and research shows that people are happiest when the person they are today is improving over the person they were yesterday.

How different would your life be if you could increase your conversion rate from 52% to over 75% or even 80%? For an office that does four new patient consultations a day, that would mean increasing from two starts a day to three. If each start adds roughly $5000 to production, it's $25,000 a week and over $1,000,000 a year. Would that help you in realizing some of your goals for your practice and the vision for your life?

If you implement the strategies I show you in this book, your office can be converting at a rate of 75-80%, as well. Throughout this book, I'll be sharing real-life examples, processes, and scripts that will get your team helping more new patients to say 'yes.'

"The Ultimate Treatment Coordinator" is my answer to your question, "How do I get more new patients?" It will answer that question and more as I show you how to implement these 5 Growth Hacks so you can hit your production goal quickly. By using the processes and scripts in this book, you and your team will be able to:

1. Respond to leads in 5 minutes or less and schedule them within 72 hours.
2. Pre-frame fees and same-day starts in the first call.
3. Double capacity with our 30-Minute New Patient Consultation.
4. Get more 'yeses' with our 5-Minute Fee Presentation.
5. Start 80% of new patients the same day with our Proven Playbook.

This book is all about sales. It's what the TC does: they're responsible for selling the treatment to the patient. I've met a lot of TCs, and they've all been great people, but the thing that all the successful practices I've worked with have in common is that their TCs are more than just salespeople: they're influencers, and I mean it in the sincerest way possible. The terms "salespeople" and "influencers," tend to turn people off because they think of the sleazy used car salesman or the superficial Instagram 'influencer' selling millions of followers products they've never even tried.

Real salespeople LOVE sales. And they do it because they genuinely love being able to give something to someone who really needs it. In fact, did you know the Latin root of the word sell, *sellar*, actually means *to give*? When you are selling someone something, you are giving them your time, knowledge, wisdom, information, and the opportunity to make an informed decision that will hopefully benefit their life.

Your TC is not trying to manipulate your patients to spend thousands of dollars on something they don't need just to make a sale. They're influencing your patients to accept and realize the person they want to be so they can help them build the bridge to get there. If a patient is feeling self-conscious about their smile, the best thing your TC can do is give them information on how they can get the smile they've always wanted. If your TC can't influence them to decide, you can't help them.

Once you get comfortable with selling, it gets really fun. Especially when you get a bonus everytime you close! My first commission sales job was at Buckle, a retail jeans store. Imagine me as a dorky teenager sizing up the girls that walked in. Once I had the whole fit thing down, I'd grab a product in her size and say, "You've gotta check out this NEW fit we have...I think you'd love it." If I could get them to try on the jeans, I could pretty much guarantee a sale. I knew exactly which fit to pull based on body type [Slim and tall are totally different than short and curvy]. If you want to be the best, you have to know everything about the product you are selling. I quickly rose to the top in sales there. I loved it because I was helping a lot of girls feel good about themselves. The added bonus is that I now know exactly how to pick out jeans for my wife!

On that note, I definitely encourage you to bonus your team members whenever they do something that increases sales or your efficiency. We're going to dig right in and get our hands dirty, deconstructing the roles on your team and redefining them so that everyone is specialized and focused on what they do best. In Chapter 1, we'll even show you a way to test your staff members' personality styles so you can make sure that they are working in their zone of genius.

People naturally resist change; it's human nature. So, in Chapter 2, I'm going to show you how to get your team opened up and receptive to change. You'll discover the 5 mindset shifts that need to happen in order to implement these 5 Growth Hacks in your practice.

Chapter 3 delivers the real goods. It shows you how to improve your whole team's efficiency with the 30-minute consultation. Best of all, it doubles your capacity for consultations, meaning you can get more new patients in sooner.

The magic happens in Chapter 4 where we go over how to present fees to make it easy for patients to say 'yes.' Get this book into your TC's hands now and have them practice using those scripts right away.

If you want to have the biggest impact on production, there is no better way to do it than by implementing the same-day start. Chapter 5 shows you the set-up and scripts you need to get new patients in your chair for bonding or iTero scanning right after the fee presentation.

Of course, not everyone is going to say 'yes' to your TC right away. Chapter 6 gives you the follow-up procedure they need to stay on top of these pending patients until they are ready to start. I'll also show you how our CRM software, PracticeBeacon (PB), can make tracking and follow up easier for your team.

In Chapter 7, I'll help you tie it all together with a walk-through, start to finish, of all these procedures and scripts so your team can visualize the entire process.

Finally, all these strategies for converting leads to new patients will have your practice growing and creating "next level" problems. While frustrating, the problems that come up are great signs of evolution. In Chapter 8, I'll show you the small, medium, and large model of orthodontic practices that can help you handle these growing pains with ease. This chapter also introduces the concepts of Book #3 of The Orthodontic Practice Growth Series, which is all about operations.

The concepts in this book are as life-changing as they are paradigm-shifting. I encourage you to ease into them with understanding and support for your team. Small changes can create big results. Remember to enjoy the process and celebrate your wins.

xx

# CHAPTER 1

# Reevaluating the Treatment Coordinator [TC] Role

*"You are out of business if you don't have a prospect."*

— Zig Zigler

When a lead comes for a new patient consultation in your office, they are taking a leap of faith. They know they want to get their crooked teeth straightened, but they are unsure about a lot of things. They don't know if they will like you, your office, or your team. They're not sure if the process will fit into their life and schedule. They're unsure about the costs and whether they can manage them. They are a lead and need to be converted into a start.

Getting more leads does not necessarily mean your practice will grow. It just means that your team has more opportunities to convert them into starts who make it into your chair. When an orthodontist says, "I just need more new patients," they don't necessarily need more leads via marketing. Often, they just need to fix their systems for conversion of the lead at the new patient consultation.

It's actually really easy to get more leads who want to fix their smiles but you have to realize that when you market online, there are three conversions that have to take place before they become a new patient.

The first conversion is getting them to respond to your marketing on your website, Facebook, or Google. Once they click through and provide their information, it's up to your scheduling coordinator to make the second conversion happen by getting a hold of the lead and scheduling a new patient consultation. The third conversion happens in the consultation room when your treatment coordinator (TC) gets the lead to agree to the fees and start treatment. If these three critical conversions do not take place, you will not be seeing that new patient in your chair.

In *Front Desk Secrets*, I refer to your scheduling coordinator as the most important and most overlooked role in your clinic. They are the interface between your community and your office. If you have a disconnect there, no amount of marketing can help you because the lead will not make it onto your schedule as a new patient consultation. You will think your marketing company is sending you bad leads, if they're even doing anything at all. For the purpose of this book, we are going to assume that your scheduling coordinators are doing a good job getting new patient consultations booked for your TC.

Let's get to it! We'll start with the premise that you've got all the new patient consultations you asked for booked into your schedule. It is now up to your TC to get that person to agree to your treatment plan and fees so they start treatment. This conversion involves the payment of $5000-$7000 paid over 24+ months. The front desk and the TC role are the most important factor and the biggest barrier to new patients getting in your chair. You definitely want to make sure you get the right people in these roles.

# Your Treatment Coordinator is Your Alchemist

Back in the 12th century, the discipline of alchemy emerged when philosophers and scientists considered the relationship between elements and the possibility of transforming an abundant, yet less valuable substance into one that was scarce and had great value. Of course, everyone was searching for a magic formula that could turn lead into gold. Your treatment coordinator is your alchemist.

Your scheduling coordinator is doing a good job if they are following up with every lead and doing everything in their power to get all viable leads booked for a new patient consultation. At the point of the consultation, those leads are only potential starts and may or may not become part of your total production. They are like a bar of lead that could be converted to gold. Your TC is the alchemist who is responsible for that conversion.

Every new patient consultation involves a person who wants a perfect smile. The question is, are they going to say 'yes' to your recommendations and accomplish that transformation with your help? Your TC is the person responsible for reassuring the new patient that they are in the right place, building trust, and getting a commitment to the treatment plan. When they do this well, the potential in that lead (no pun intended) becomes realized and they become a start, adding $5,000 to $7,000 to production. It's almost magical, isn't it?

While a formula for transforming lead into gold was never discovered, we do know that there are some TCs who have the magic touch that can take almost any lead, turn them into a new patient, and increase production. They perform the new patient consultation, interact with the doctor, make sure the new patient understands treatment, sort out payment of fees, and get them in the chair the same day. It's astonishing, and you want to set them up so they can do that all day, every day. There is a formula for this and we are going to make sure you understand it and can replicate it with your TC in your office by the end of this book.

If you want your TC to be an alchemist, you must set up some very important conditions for their success:

1. You must find **the right person for the TC role** (Not everyone can be an alchemist).
2. The scheduling coordinator must provide them with the right starting material in the form of **pre-qualified and pre-framed leads.**
3. **Don't interfere while they're working their magic** (In a lot of cases, the more the doctor talks in the consultation, the less likely new patients are to commit to treatment and make a down payment).
4. **Recognize and reward their value** (Make the TC role a dedicated position and bonus them for performance).

All magic aside, turning a lead from Facebook or Google into a $5,000-$7,000 same day start in your chair within 72 hours is a sales process.

## The TC is in Sales

As healthcare providers, it's hard to wrap your head around the fact that you work in sales, but that's the reality. Most orthodontists just wish that they had patients showing up in their chair so they could help as many people in their community as possible. Sadly, this can't happen without sales. If the patient does not agree to the treatment and payment terms, they will not start and you don't get to help them.

The discussion of fees can be one of the easiest things to get right, however, in most offices, it usually goes horribly wrong. Talking money is somewhat taboo and no one really loves blurting out, "Treatment will be SIX THOUSAND DOLLARS," but sadly, this is exactly what is done. The prospect is left thinking, "OMG, how am I going to afford this?" or, "How am I going to pitch this to dad?" Fortunately, there is an easy script that will keep this conversation from blowing them out of the water. The fourth growth hack, our five-minute fee presentation, is covered in Chapter 4.

In most offices we work with, everyone seems to dance around the fact that we must get a commitment out of these new patients for large sums of money. They hope that the person thinks the staff is nice enough, the orthodontist is smart enough, and they want a great smile badly enough to just glance over the fees and hopefully get a 'yes.' Fortunately, people do want straight teeth and the fact that they came into your office is a testament to that. Because a smile is so valued in our culture, the average conversion rate across the country is 52%. This happens even if your TC is bad at selling.

The magic happens when we embrace the fact that we are in business and we have to get well trained in sales. Why are one in two people in your office saying 'no' to a process that they have already told you they want? Could your sales process be part of the problem? Is your office making it difficult for a person who is unhappy with the state of their teeth to commit to a process they want and need? The answer is 'yes!' TCs who are skilled in the art of sales are converting at a rate over 80%. The best TCs are getting 80% of those people who say 'yes' into their orthodontist's chair that same day.

However, not everyone is cut out for sales. Some people are just better suited to other roles and that's okay. We all have different personality styles and they predispose us to our likes and dislikes. Some love interacting with people whereas others are happier focusing on tasks. Some enjoy influencing people while others are stimulated by solving problems. That's why it pays to find the right person who can be an alchemist in the TC role. Someone who can become the ultimate salesperson who inspires new patients to take action today to get the smile they want in the next 12 to 24 months.

## 1. The Right Person for the TC Role

Not everyone on your team can do this. When you are hiring TCs, you should be looking for outgoing, people-oriented, and influential candidates. They should be enthusiastic, extroverted, and lively when communicating. They must look forward to engaging and interacting with your patients and impacting their lives. This can be hard to determine after just one interview with an applicant, and sometimes, it takes a while for people to come out of their shells and show their true colors.

I asked Vanessa Fitzwater, the Treatment Coordinator from Knecht Orthodontics, why she's been so successful in the TC role over these last few years. Here's what she had to say:

"I could talk to a brick wall. I'm definitely an outgoing person, for sure. To do this job, you have to be a people person and you need to know how to read people. So even though I can talk about anything, I have to gauge how the person is first. Some patients are more quiet and reserved, so I'm not going to talk their ear off. But some patients come in and want to know your life story. So it's knowing how to interact with these different personalities. When you come across many different types of people every day, you can practice and eventually get used to it. But even in scenarios where people are more reserved, you still have to be a people person—you want to try to get them out of their shell so they can trust you."

## The Predictive Index

A great way to determine if someone is the right fit for the TC role is by having them take a psychometric test as a part of their interview process. For example, The Predictive Index (PI) offers psychometrics testing specifically targeted at businesses to help them find the right employees to fill roles. The PI assessments help them understand the needs of a role, team, project, or business strategy, as well as collect and use candidate or employee data to make more informed decisions about who to hire and how to manage.

However, these aren't actual "tests" that the individual passes or fails. It really just provides an overview of who they are as a person, and you can decide if they fit the roles they're trying to fill. Businesses can use their Job Assessment feature to analyze each role and identify the underlying traits a candidate should have to be successful in the role. Then, when they need to hire, they can have candidates complete their Behavioral and Cognitive Assessments, which will help measure each candidate's behavioral drives and cognitive ability. These are quick tests, so they won't take up too much time for candidates to complete (the Behavioral Assessment takes 6 minutes, and the Cognitive Assessment takes 12 minutes). The business receives a report that provides attributes of the candidate's personality, and from there, they can determine if the candidate is the right fit.

Can you really know someone's true personality after only taking 20 minutes worth of assessments? Not entirely, but you'll have a good idea. The PI groups different personalities into a series of Profiles, such as the Analytical Profile, Persistent Profile, Social Profile, and Stabilizing Profile. So, if you look at different job assessments, you'll be able to understand which profile best fits the job description and it'll be easier to narrow down the hiring process.

I actually used their Job Assessment feature to determine the attributes and characteristics of the TC role, and the results substantiated my hypothesis. Based on their description, the TC role should be fulfilled by someone who portrays one of the following traits from the Social Profile:

1. The Persuader: Someone who is a risk-taker, is socially poised, and motivated to build teams.

2. The Captain: Someone who is a problem solver, likes change and innovation, and enjoys controlling the big picture.

3. The Promoter: Someone who is casual, informal, expressive, persuasive, and extroverted.

Personalities that fall within the Social Profile are suitable for roles involving sales. If you'd like to learn more about the different profiles outlined by the Predictive Index, scan this QR code.

Madison Martin, the Director of Sales at Fishbein Orthodontics, gladly volunteered to take the Predictive Index's Behavioral Assessment and allowed us to highlight her results in this book.

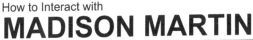

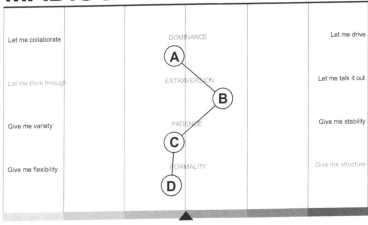

How to Interact with
# MADISON MARTIN
Promoter

| Let me collaborate | | DOMINANCE | | | Let me drive |
| Let me think through | | EXTRAVERSION | | | Let me talk it out |
| Give me variety | | PATIENCE | | | Give me stability |
| Give me flexibility | | FORMALITY | | | Give me structure |

A
B
C
D

PI THE PREDICTIVE INDEX

© Predictive Index, LLC 1995 – 2022

Learn more about The Predictive Index at www.predictiveindex.com

Scan this QR code to view Madison's complete PI Behavioral Report.

SCAN ME

While the report provides a detailed analysis of the subject's personality, let's look at how this assessment identifies the traits that make her such an ideal fit for the TC role:

## Strongest Behaviors

While moderate, Madison will most strongly express the following behaviors:

- Relatively informal and outgoing with others. Communicates in an open, lively, flexible manner, drawing others into the conversation.
- More interested in people, building relationships, and teamwork than technical matters. Generally affable, optimistic, and trusting.
- More focused on goals and the people needed to get there than the details or plans; comfortable delegating details.
- Socially-focused, generally empathizes with people, seeing their point of view or understanding their emotions. Positive communication.
- Teaches and shares; generally interested in working collaboratively with others to help out.
- Friendly and service-oriented; drives for the "greater good" rather than individual goals. Promotes teamwork by sharing authority.
- Relatively quick in connecting to others; reasonably open and sharing. Builds and leverages relationships to get work done.
- Fluent, enthusiastic, and comparatively frequent in communication; a motivator who pays attention to others' points of view.
- Collaborative; works with and through others. Focused on team cohesion, dynamics, and interpersonal relations.

Reading through Madison's behaviors, it's immediately quite obvious why she thrives in the role of Director of Sales at Fishbein Orthodontics. She is a good communicator who builds rapport quickly and makes people feel at ease. She can get people focused on the big picture goal of creating the great smile they crave without diving down the rabbit hole of how that's going to happen. The orthodontist and assistants are there to make that happen. What's important to her is the person right in front of her. She connects to them with empathy for their situation and helps to engage them in the process of creating results. People want to be part of her team and find it easy to say 'yes' to the plan that she presents.

# SUMMARY:

Madison is an outgoing, talkative, very friendly individual, and a lively and stimulating communicator. A good mixer who is poised, active and responsive in social situations.

The complete extrovert; informal and uninhibited in their behavior; understand people well and is capable of using that understanding to gain the friendship and cooperation of others. It is important to these individuals to be liked and accepted, and they express themself to individuals or groups with warmth and enthusiasm. Easily understands and accepts other viewpoints, ideas, and feelings, and can be effective at getting diverse groups to come together and collaborate.

Relatively unconcerned about details and often inclined to consider them unimportant, this individual expresses themself in general terms, aimed more at gaining the interest or attention of others than at communicating specific, factual information. Their interest in details and specifics which are not crucial to success is, at best, casual. As such, they focus on the "big picture" personal goals, and if appropriate, their colleagues, direct reports, or team. They're flexible about how they attain these goals, often thinking "out of the box" and collaborating widely to get there. Their work pace is faster-than-average and they can learn quickly, but rather generally, if left on their own. Because of their strong social orientation, group learning, mentors, and coaches are most effective.

Cheerful and upbeat; makes friends easily and enjoys doing things for people, although they're rather casual about exactly how things are done. This individual's friendly, enthusiastic style makes others feel welcome. Strongly persuasive; has complete confidence in their ability to gain others' trust and buy-in; is persistent and won't take "no" for an answer.

The last three paragraphs of this summary of Madison's personality highlight why she is the perfect person for helping new patients become starts. Her casual attitude, fast pace, and "out of the box" thinking make it easy for her to respond to a person's concerns on the fly to come up with a payment plan that works for them. Because she is so friendly and empathetic, people find her persistence helpful rather than pushy.

Another of our clients had two staff members who would alternate between assisting the orthodontist and the TC role. When I looked at their conversion rates, I found that one was closing 15% more than the other. When I looked into this further, the TC with the higher conversion rate enjoyed the TC role more than assisting. The TC with the lower conversion rate preferred assisting. If we take a look at her Predictive Index, you can see why she is more partial to a more stable, predictable, and technical assistant role.

How to Interact with
# JOANNE WINTERS

Craftsman

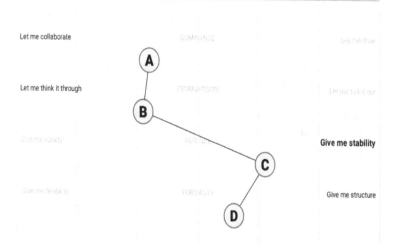

## Strongest Behaviors

Joanne will most strongly express the following behaviors:

- Private, serious, introspective, and reserved. Takes time to connect to and trust new people.
- Focused; can concentrate on the task at hand for long periods. Quickly notices and understands technical matters more than social ones. Consistent and patiently thoughtful.
- Works at a steady, unwavering pace; most comfortable with familiar processes, environments, and co-workers. Doesn't easily change.
- Unhurried and deliberate, stable and will do things using the established process; it is difficult to change these systems. Dependable, consistent and needs familiar environments and coworkers to be most productive.
- Cooperative, easy-going, and agreeable in getting along with others. A focused, uncritical listener who won't "rock the boat."
- Methodical, steady, and even-paced; loses productivity when interrupted.
- Formal, reserved, introspective, and skeptical of new people; requires "proof" to build trust in new people.
- Detail-oriented and precise; follow-through is deep and literal to ensure tasks were completed in accordance with quality standards.
- Operationally, as opposed to socially, focused. Thinks, in specific terms, about what needs to be done and how to do it accurately and flawlessly; follows, in a literal way, that execution plan.

This is quite a contrast to Madison's profile so you can see why you may want to think twice about engaging Joanne for the role of TC. The demands of the TC role would place a lot of stress on this staff person and leave them in a far from resourceful state. Joanne was very happy when she was moved to the assistant role permanently.

# Summary

Joanne is thoughtful, disciplined, and particularly attentive to, careful of, and accurate with the details involved in the job. Identifies problems, and enjoys solving them, particularly within their area of expertise. Works at a steady, even pace, leveraging their background for the betterment of the team, company, or customer.

With experience and/or training, they will develop a high level of specialized expertise. Serious and dedicated to the job and the company. Their work pace is steady and even-keeled, and they're motivated by a real concern for getting work done thoroughly and correctly. Discipline and circumspect thinking will lend caution to their decision-making; Joanne plans ahead, double checks, and follows up carefully on decisions and actions.

A modest and unassuming person, they work autonomously in their area of expertise. When working outside of that area, their drive is to seek specialized knowledge by finding definitive answers from written resources, authoritative management, or established subject-matter experts. Is most effective and productive when they work within or close to their specialty and experience, and prefer to stick to the proven way. If it becomes necessary for to initiate or adopt change, Joanne will need to see cold, hard, evidence to prove that the new way is proven, complete, and yields high-quality results. In addition, they'll carefully plan the implementation to minimize problems and maximize results.

This individual is reserved and accommodating, expressing themself sincerely and factually. In general, they're rather cautious and conservative in style, skeptical about anything new or unfamiliar or any change in the traditional way of doing things. Possessing the ability to strongly concentrate on the job at hand, they are most effective when given uninterrupted blocks of time. Has better-than-average aptitude for work that is analytical or technical in nature.

Joanne's personality style is not bad, it's just not best suited to the TC role. She is now thriving in the assistant role because she is not having her steadiness disrupted by the stress of alternating jobs. Because she can count on the stability of performing the same technical work on a daily basis, she can focus on refining her skills and becoming more knowledgeable about the details of the processes.

If you do decide to use a personality assessment, such as the Predictive Index, to determine a candidate's suitability for a particular role, remember that it is just a starting point. It can help you to determine if they will be a good fit in a sales-oriented role like the TC or the scheduling coordinator. If they have a more introverted, detail-oriented style, they will likely do better in a more technical, process-oriented role in your clinic.

Ultimately, not everyone is cut out for the TC role. If you want to have a TC who is an alchemist, turning all your viable leads into starts, then make sure you hire the right person for the job. Once you have this person in the TC role, it is imperative that they be given the right starting materials if you want to see conversion and increased production. This means that your scheduling coordinators must set the TC up for success by pre-qualifying and pre-framing the lead.

If you'd like to work with someone to build out roles, profiles, and an org chart for your practice, as well as recruit the best candidates, I would contact Wiseman Strategies. You can listen to my podcast with their team by scanning the QR code.

## 2. Pre-qualified and Pre-framed Leads

In order to ensure the sale will go smoothly, your front desk and scheduling coordinators must play a consistent role in the set up. Teamwork during this process is essential, so everyone has to pull their weight for the new patient consultation to convert effectively. The goal of the scheduling coordinator is to take those leads that say they're interested, and pre-qualify, pre-frame, and schedule them within 72 hours of initial contact. This gives the TC the perfect starting material to transform that lead into a same-day start.

If your scheduling coordinators are top-notch, they've already debriefed the full consultation, telling your prospective patients what to expect, the average fees for treatment, and advising them about the possibility and convenience of a same-day start if the doctor thinks they're ready. They should have also sent the patient all the paperwork they need to fill out before their appointment with the TC in the welcome email. All these steps save time during the new patient consultations and pre-frame the patient so they are not surprised by fees or questioning whether they should start treatment right away. The patients have a transparent, efficient, and enjoyable consultation and your TC has an easier time convincing them that they are in the right place and ready to commit to treatment.

Beverly Simkins, the Lead Front Desk and Scheduling Coordinator at Cassinelli, Shaker, and Baker Orthodontics, also has years of experience as a TC, so she knows what to look out for to set them up for success:

"I always check to see if the patient included their dentist's information so I can reach out to them to see if there are any current x-rays. We don't have to take x-rays during the consultation if there are. If the x-rays aren't current, we will take them and even send those x-rays to their dentist so they don't need to do them again. Patients appreciate that, but so do our TCs, as it shaves time off their consultations. I also do the same thing with insurance. Validating insurance can take some time, so I always try to get their insurance information before their *appointment. All I have to do is send it to our financial coordinator and determine if insurance will cover part of the treatment. It's taken care of before they arrive at their consultation."*

Paperwork can be pretty time-consuming, so having them complete the 6 pages of paperwork at home makes the consultation walkthrough relatively easy. They just have to check in at the front desk, go through the records process with the records technician, have a brief discussion with the doctor, and discuss treatment and fees with the TC. If your scheduling coordinator walks through everything correctly in the initial conversation, the patient already knows about the same-day start option so that when the TC brings it up, they feel at ease to get started right away.

## 3. Don't Interfere While They're Working Their Magic

Setting the TC up for success not only involves helping them to do a better job but also giving them the space to do what they do best. This is such an important role that you must make sure they are not distracted by other responsibilities, like working the front desk or assisting the orthodontist. As you'll see in the next chapter, you want them ready and focused for the next new patient consultation which will be happening in 30 minutes.

You'll also see how critical it is that the doctor trusts that the TC has the conversion of the new patient handled. Spending more time trying to explain everything that is going on with their teeth decreases the chances of them starting the same day. Get in and meet the patient. Give them your recommendations and get out in two minutes or less.

## 4. Recognize and Reward Their Value

The personality styles that do well in the TC role thrive on recognition and will work harder to hit goals if rewards are involved. We interviewed several TCs for this book. When I asked them what motivates them to excel in their role, each TC had the same response: "I'm motivated by bonuses and incentives!" When your TC is doing everything they can to get every new patient to same-day start, they are making you money. It goes without saying that you should share the wealth. It creates great morale and builds an innovative team that strives to constantly improve.

## Maintaining Excellent Customer Service

Not every appointment is straightforward. Doctors and TCs see a lot of different cases during these exams daily, and unfortunately, there are times when the patient cannot start treatment right away. For example, some patients need to see a dentist before starting orthodontic treatment. Beverly recounts a severe case she once witnessed:

> "One time, we had a woman come in who desperately wanted braces, but after going through the consultation and examining her records, we quickly realized she couldn't be a candidate since her teeth were so fragile. The prospective patient revealed that she never went to the dentist and didn't take very good care of her teeth. In her case, we referred her to a dentist for dental work. I don't know if she'll ever qualify for orthodontic care based on the status of her teeth, but sometimes these are the types of cases you get, and you have to turn them down and do your best to provide them with the proper referrals so they can still receive quality care. We can't do anything for her until all of that is taken care of."

In these cases, it's essential to be transparent with the patient and give them the proper referrals to improve their oral health, as that's ultimately the most important thing. TCs need to be compassionate in these situations. It's not always about making a sale but acting with integrity. If you know the prospective patient isn't a candidate for treatment at this time, they need to know that. The patients will appreciate the honesty and will most likely seek your services in the future once they've addressed the concerns you and your team have outlined for them.

It goes without saying that providing outstanding customer service to patients as a TC is crucial. A good mindset for a TC to have to ensure they are doing everything in their power to encourage a patient to same-day start without being pushy is "committed but not attached." This means they have the patient's best interest at heart and are invested in helping them to make a decision that will improve their lives but do not care what decision the patient makes either way. Therefore, the patient feels their empathy, compassion, and concern rather than their desire to close this sale to get a bonus.

While closing the sale is their primary goal, TCs should provide optimum patient care beyond just trying to get them to start. This includes being transparent, friendly, and supportive while providing effective communication inside and outside the office via follow-up and reminder calls, emails, and text messages to all current and prospective patients.

Beverly continues to maintain excellent relationships with her patients. She recalls a moment when she was in the TC role that stuck with her:

> "I try to build a rapport with my patients. I actually had one patient's mom call me what felt like 5 million times, asking me questions about everything. She was super nice, and I tried to be as helpful as possible to ease her anxieties. One day the patient and his mom came in. He came right up to me and said, "Ms. Bev, do not talk money with my mom until you get the insurance straightened out because she'll say no to me getting braces." The mom chimes in and says, "He's not wrong." We all ended up laughing so hard.

*The insurance ended up covering a huge part of the fees, so the patient started treatment. He came in a few weeks later, ran up to me and gave me a big hug, and said, "Ms. Bev, what's going on? Thank you so much for doing what you did, or my mom would have said no." That one experience was the foundation of our great dynamic now. I try to make sure I do what I can to help patients out and make light of situations when things get a bit tough."*

The bottom line is this: if your team members are in positions where they need to interact with the public daily, they need to be great at providing customer service. If they can't do it right, they shouldn't be doing it. This is just as important as selling. They need to keep it light and make it convenient for the patient. They need to influence, not push. They need to act with integrity and empathy, always. And if the patient decides to start treatment, let your TC know they can give them a small thank you gift. If they decide not to start today, the TC should continue to follow up with them—every single time.

## Change Happens One Step at a Time

If reading this chapter makes you think, I've got to make some changes here, write down a few goals and share them with your team. Perhaps it's time to share this book with them, as well. Maybe this chapter has sparked some light bulbs and given you ideas that will make your team more effective. Perhaps it is showing you that the way you have always thought things worked is not the only way. Wherever you are in your journey, following in the footsteps of people who are getting the results that you want will help get you there. If your mind is simply having trouble processing some of the concepts that I have just shared, read on. In the next chapter, we will address the mindset shifts that need to happen in order for you and your team to grow to new levels.

# CHAPTER 2
# Fostering the Right Mindset

*"Progress is impossible without change and those who cannot change their minds cannot change anything."*

— George Bernard Shaw

The one thing we can always count on in life is change. It's funny because change is also the one thing that people seem to be most resistant to. However, no matter how stuck we are in our ways, the world around us will eventually force us to do something different. If you're reading this book, it's because you want a different result in your office. You want to be able to see more new patients so you can grow your practice, help more people, and have financial freedom. Whatever your reasons for wanting to grow your practice, growth requires us to look at things differently and do things that we have never done before. When we are faced with new challenges and possibilities we often run into the biggest obstacle of them all: ourselves.

When Dr. Ben Fishbein from Fishbein Orthodontics first opened his practice back in 2013, it was not run the way it currently is in 2022. Dr. Fishbein spent a lot of time doing everything himself, and eventually realized it was only hindering the growth of the practice. He realized he needed to hire people to fulfill these roles so that he could focus on just being the doctor:

> "*In the very early stages, when I was working, I was hustling. I was going to every dental office, doing any kind of marketing I could that didn't require a lot of money because I didn't have it. Lots of boots-on-the-ground stuff... But if you want to grow, you have to hire, even if you're taking a cut on your margins. It's better to be overstaffed than understaffed... When you fast forward to today, I'm just seeing patients and helping out with the management. Everyone on my team has a specialized role that helps contribute to the growth of the practice.*"

If you want your TC to thrive in the vision you have for your practice, you need to inspire them to change how they see their role and their interactions with people daily. It begins with a subtle shift in mindset for both you and your TC and you must lead by example to create buy-in.

## Mindset Shift #1: The TC Role is a Specialized Role

When I first start working with an office, I find all sorts of scenarios. 90% of offices have a TC in some way, shape, or form. In about 5% of cases, we've found a doctor doing the TC role which is a terrible idea if you want to scale. In 50-60% of the cases, the person in the TC role is also performing other roles like the front desk or clinical assistant. Which leaves 20-30% of offices where the TC is a dedicated role and the person is only focused on one thing: turning new patients into starts.

> "*A jack of all trades, but a master of none.*"

If you have read Front Desk Secrets, you will notice that we are into the specialization of roles at HIP. We find it much more efficient to have a team member highly trained and immersed in one part of the operation than to jump around fulfilling a number of different tasks and duties.
It's common for businesses to hire employees to fill one role and then expect them to wear many hats within that role.

While this approach forces the employee to learn how to do a bunch of different tasks, they usually end up doing a sub-par job at each task because they haven't dedicated enough time and effort to it. It's not their fault. It's very difficult to thrive in a role when you are being pulled in multiple directions and expected to complete unrelated tasks.

For this reason, the TC role in your practice needs to be specialized. Your TC should be responsible for only one thing: selling the treatment plan to your new patients. Yes, there are a lot of different tasks they have to do to achieve this, but they are different from having to answer the phone, respond to email requests for appointments, or check patients in at the front desk. Providing the best service to the patient must be their only focus so they can ultimately sell your treatment plan and add $5000-$7000 to production. We don't want them feeling overworked, underappreciated, and burnt out.

Specialization of roles based on personality will result in happier employees, better workplace morale, and a practice that runs like a well-oiled machine. Everyone needs to know their role and stay in their lane, while at the same time understand the need for teamwork and collaboration.

## Mindset Shift #2: The Patient is Pre-Sold

If a patient shows up to your office for a free consultation, there are a number of things that we can deduce:

1. Their teeth are crooked and they are insecure about their smile.
2. They are motivated to take action to build a better smile.
3. They are considering your clinic as the place to do it.
4. They have already invested the time and energy to get to your office.
5. They have taken a leap of faith to embark on what they

know will be an expensive and long-term process. These things all stack up in your favor when pre-qualifying them for the close. The only things left to find out are whether they have the financial means of moving forward and if they are willing to do what it takes to follow the treatment protocol at your clinic.

Let's make the assumption that they can in fact afford one of your payment plans and their desire to look better is strong enough that they will make the time to follow your recommendations. If these factors turn out to be true, there should be no reason for them to decline starting care. To put it simply, the patient is pre-closed until proven otherwise.

This is the mindset that I want shaping your attitude towards every new patient that enters your office. When your behavior comes from your belief that these people are here to get in the chair today, you'll find that you'll be taking credit cards and escorting them back to get started almost every time. This is the type of thinking that moves your conversion rate from the national average of one in two to the exceptional close rate of three out of four. That's an increase from 52% to over 75%. Many TCs I've worked with are now converting at a rate over 80%.

There are some obstacles that can sometimes get in the way of making this an instant reality. I like to call these things objections. When people start giving objections about why they can't do something, our first instinct is to counter them. But that only causes their guards to go up even higher, and eventually, you'll end up losing them.

Our guards are always up when we are unsure or don't have enough information to make an informed decision about something. To avoid this, you need to ensure your TC knows how to eliminate objections from the beginning so that they don't occur. To do this successfully, they must be clear and transparent from the start. We will cover the four objections that you must pre-emptively eliminate every time to ensure a smooth close in Chapter 4.

## Mindset Shift #3: Gain Certainty from the Truth, the Facts, and the Reality

Whenever I find myself in an uncertain situation, I like to build up my certainty by asking myself three questions:

1. What is the truth?
2. What are the facts?
3. What is the reality?

The truth is the concept that must be true in order for me to get the outcome I want in a particular situation. In the case of closing a patient in the TC consultation, I want the patient to agree to the fees and treatment plan and get in the chair today. In this case, we know the truth is that this person wants their teeth straightened, otherwise they would not seek out a free consultation at an orthodontist's office.

The facts are the evidence that you can find to support the truth that you require in order to get the outcome you want. The facts are that the patient came to your office for a reason; they came to find certainty and hopefully get a treatment plan to start their smile journey. If you want this new patient to agree to start today, you just need to check off the list of the five facts that would make them pre-sold above.

The reality is simply the situation that I find myself in that is posing uncertainty. When I can state out loud for myself what that reality is, it becomes something that I can troubleshoot and resolve. In this case, it comes down to human nature and the fact that everyone is guarded when they enter a new situation with people they don't know or trust yet. We are asking them to make a big decision that involves a lot of money and a huge commitment. It's understandable that they are guarded.

## Mindset Shift #4: I Am a Guard-Disarming Agent

How do we get people to lower their guard? We need to become guard-disarming agents. Words have power. A subtle change in our language when conversing with patients is all it takes to see those guards drop. We covered techniques and phrases that you can use to help people drop their defenses in *Front Desk Secrets*, the first book of this series. Let's review them here.

Below are two statements that basically say the same thing, however there are subtle differences in tone:

- We do offer same-day starts... so, that means we can start treatment today if you are interested.
- We do offer same-day starts, so that means you are able to start treatment today if that might possibly be convenient for you? How does that sound?

The first statement abruptly gets right to it, whereas the second statement is a little wordier, but for a good reason. It uses softer language and feels non-threatening; it's positioned as though you are putting the ball in their court to decide what works best for them. Softening words such as might, maybe, possibly, and convenient can transform a statement that seems pushy and abrupt into one that relays the same message in a way that feels like it's their idea.

You can also use connecting phrases to make the message more meaningful to the patient. Examples of connecting phrases include: so that you can...; in order to... which will allow you to...; which means you...; etc. [A list of these phrases and how to use them can be found in *Front Desk Secrets*].

Take a look at this example:

- We can offer you a same-day start so you can start treatment without having to come in for another appointment, which means you won't have to take more time off work, if that might possibly be convenient for you?

By using both connecting phrases and softening words, we continuously position and frame the interaction in a way that saves them time and offers them convenience. Ultimately, people really only care about one thing: what's in it for them.

This is not only important for your TC but for all public and patient-facing roles in your office. I recommend doing a training with these softening words and connecting phrases with your team. Work through the different types of interactions that happen in your office where people may be guarded. Find the opportunities to soften the dialogue and role play the scenarios until the wording becomes second nature.

## Mindset Shift #5: Capacity for Consultations

The capacity that an orthodontist has for consultations is one of the biggest limiting factors to the growth of a clinic. It has been standard practice in the industry to do one-hour consultations with the orthodontist spending 20-30 minutes in the room with the new patient. We have seen some doctors who spend up to 60 minutes in a new patient consultation before they have even committed to start treatment. This means that in an eight-hour work day, many clinics only have the capacity to see maybe six or seven new patient consultations if we allow an hour for lunch. This is also assuming they have a very light load in the clinic. If they are slammed seeing established patients, they may only have time for 2-3 new patient consults.

If your scheduling coordinators can book more consultations in a day, your TC will have more opportunities to convert new patients into starts. That's a fact. But with this mindset shift, everyone in the office has to believe it to become real. That means the scheduling coordinators should be booking more leads for consultations with your TC, the record technicians must be taking records quickly, the TC should be efficiently going through the treatment and fee presentation, and the orthodontist pops in only briefly to introduce themself and deliver the treatment plan. A team effort is required for this to work smoothly, or there will be hitches and the whole system will be inclined to revert to a lower capacity.

When I start working with a new practice, I always have to wrestle with them to get them to consider reducing their new patient consultation time. When I ask them why they feel they need to do 60-minute consultations with new patients, I always hear that they need the time to create a relationship with their patients and don't want them to feel rushed.

Now I'm sure you're all very nice people and your friends think you're great, but do you really think this new patient who has never met you, is not sure if they trust you and is hesitant about whether your clinic is the right choice, really wants to hang out with you longer than they need to? I've been around thousands of orthodontists and in my experience, many of them are much more comfortable chairside, doing their thing or talking shop with other doctors, describing weird and wonderful teeth rotations that they have corrected. Trust me. The average person does not care to hear the gory details of what's going on in their mouth. All they want to know is if you can fix it, how long it will take, and how much it will cost them. Why don't you leave the customer service to the friendlier and bubblier team members?

Kasey Workman, the Lead Treatment Coordinator at Fishbein Orthodontics, explains how her office eventually went from the 60-minute consultation to the 30-minute consultation:

> "We slowly got into the process of 30-minute consultations. When I first started, we had an hour per consultation. Then Dr. Fishbein decided that we were going to do 45 minutes, so to do that, we just slowly had to get quicker with each step of our process. Then one day, he decided it would be 30 minutes. So the doctors need to understand that to make that happen, they have to do their part; they can't spend 20 minutes of our 30-minutes in the room. So they're very quick; the doctors trust the TCs because they know what they're talking about: they know how to explain the treatment to the patient. They also know if the patient has more questions, you can go grab the doctor again, but that never happens."

Your practice should aim to cut that 60-minute consultation in half. This shift in mindset has to happen for everyone on your team. It's a process and the change will not happen overnight. If you're wondering how you can implement this, I'll tell you in detail in the next chapter.

## Mindset Shift #6: Incentives for TCs

We've already pre-framed the fact that you need to consider your TC as the top salesperson with the power to influence people to make decisions to change their lives for the better; to bring them from uncertain to certain; to help them cross that bridge from who they currently are to the person they want to become. Great! This is a powerful role they have been given, and just like all top performing salespeople, they need to be rewarded when their efforts are successful.

Unfortunately, not many practices reward their TCs when sales are made. The mindset shift is that the more the TC closes, the more money I make, therefore it makes sense to incentivize my TC to do everything in their power to close the sale. Think about it. If your TC is getting paid the same amount whether they close eight starts or none at all, what is their motivation to go above and beyond to make sure each and every new patient can say 'yes' to starting care? On top of that, if they're doing the math and adding up all the money they are bringing into the practice yet they are not getting any appreciation or compensation for doing so, they're going to get resentful. Their morale will start to drop and their close rate will decrease even faster. They will stop caring, and the new patients will feel it and leave your office looking for a more positive place to spend $5000-$7000.

When salespeople know they are rewarded for selling, they perform at a higher level. Time and again, we've seen incentives work magic for orthodontic staff members. When your team is rewarded for the practice's performance, every team member pulls together to help make your business grow. As a result, your revenue and profits also grow. More importantly, your patients feel the positive energy and motivation of the team members. It creates an extraordinary environment that makes patients excited to start treatment with you.

If you aren't currently providing bonuses to the team members that help you reach your goals, you need to implement a rewards structure ASAP. Not an across-the-board bonus to everyone whenever your sales increase, but a specific, measurable bonus that motivates each person to perform their role better. When they hit their target, they get the reward.

Dr. Ben Fishbein likes to say, "Bonus the behaviors you want to see more of." His offices have a great culture full of excited staff members who are committed to growth.

Kasey reveals how the commission-based structure at Fishbein Orthodontics has been paramount for TCs in their office:

*"Our TCs are all commission-based, so they are so motivated to get everyone in for a same-day start. They get bonuses on same-day starts, selling the retainer plan, and selling the Zoom whitening. It's really made us happier to come to work, and it pushes us to work harder and smarter to get that commission check every time."*

In addition to a commission-based structure, you can also create office-wide contests to keep everyone on their toes! It may be less practical to give bonuses to all of your team members, but the front desk and scheduling coordinators, records technicians, and other staff all play a part in getting the patient started for treatment. One way to motivate them is to set up a weekly or monthly contest to incentivize whatever goal you're trying to reach. It could be a number of new patient starts, several same-day starts, the speed of the record techs, or even successfully booking new exams within 72 hours. After all, accomplishing everything in this book will require some changes in processes and behaviors at your office. Giving incentives is the most effective way to get your team to commit to the significant changes you'll need to make to start closing patients more effectively.

## Change Your Thoughts, Change Your Life

All it really takes to get you from where you are today to where you dream of being is a few mindset shifts. If you aren't willing to change your perspectives about how to run your office, change will happen very slowly, if at all. As the leader of your team, you need to set the standards for what is possible. You must motivate and inspire them to be positive and work hard. You need to buy into an idea first before you can expect your team to get on board. The mindset shifts discussed in this chapter will put your office into a state of growth. Once the entire team has adopted these perspectives, it will feel like nothing can stop the success and growth of your practice.

Now that you know the headspace that's necessary to experience rapid growth, let's move on to how you can wow new patients, create trust and connection, and convert more of them into starts with the 30-Minute Consultation.

# CHAPTER 3

# Implementing the 30-Minute Consultation

*"Your excuses might be legit, but they won't improve your life."*

— Grant Cardone

In order to grow your practice, you will need to see more patients. The first question you should be asking yourself is whether your current systems can handle more new patient exams. Does increased volume mean you have to work longer hours? Will you need to hire more staff to handle the flow necessary to support growth? Is your team even ready for this or will they get flustered, drop balls, and drive new patients away?

Most of the time, when doctors hire marketing companies to increase the number of new patients, we see that they have no idea how to turn the leads into new patient consultations. The staff aren't ready for an increase in patient volume and they remain stuck at their current practice volume. It's as if practice volume is a setting on a thermostat.

When you set your thermostat to maintain the room temperature at 70 degrees, it makes adjustments to restore the preset temperature whenever the temperature moves up or down. If the room gets too cold, the heat comes on to bring the temperature back up to 70. If the room temperature rises above 70, the air conditioning turns on to bring it back down.

No matter what, unless you change the preset temperature, the thermostat will keep the room at 70 degrees.

You and your team, your mindset, systems, and procedures are a set point that maintains your practice volume where it is. When things slow down, you hustle to get more patient visits booked. If the days start getting a little hectic, people start to drop balls, let things slide, and the pace slows back to the setpoint.

If you want to increase your practice volume, you need to adjust the setpoint of your practice. Otherwise, when you turn on the marketing to increase the volume, that thermostat will just cool things down and you will be frustrated by the dollars you wasted on marketing for no results.

If you and your team take the time to implement all the mindset shifts from the last chapter, you will be well on your way to adjusting your office setpoint to handle a much higher volume of patients. The chapters that follow will show you the systems and processes that you need to put in place so that your team can convert the influx of leads from marketing campaigns into new patient consultations and then to starts without leaking out or breaking the system.

The first thing that we need to do is create the capacity for the inflow of new patients. We absolutely must shorten the length of a new patient consultation if we want to fit more into our day without having to work longer hours. In this chapter, I am going to show you how the nations top 1% orthodontic practices run 30-minute consultations to provide ample capacity for new patients and growth.

Here's the secret formula:

- 8 minutes for the records technician.
- 2-5 minutes for the doctor's consultation.
- 5 minutes for the TC's fee presentation.

Here is a visual timeline:

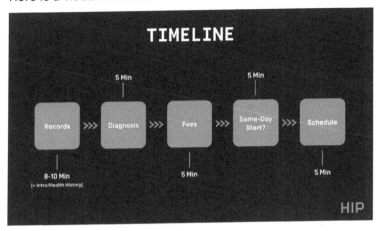

Wait! What? That's only 15-30 minutes! I can already hear some of you saying, "There's no way!" I also know that every great idea has been first met with great resistance.

Don't worry. I'm not saying that you and your team need to try to make this a reality in your office tomorrow. Of course you're going to need to wrap your head around the concept and get your team on board with making the changes necessary to perform a comprehensive consultation this quickly while delivering extraordinary patient care.

"But Luke, you said it was a 30-minute consultation. Where are the other 15 minutes?" When you get each consult down like this every time, the extra 15 minutes can be used for check-in, paperwork, the office tour, and scheduling the start date, which will hopefully take place that same day.

Before we get into the specifics of how to do this, let's get Kasey from Fishbein Orthodontics to walk us through how this works in their office. Keep in mind that they have multiple doctors and TCs working in eight locations:

"We have 30 minutes total with each patient, so we typically schedule up to 33 or more a day. The patient will arrive and the first step is to fill out paperwork. We always try to reduce that step by having them fill it out online before their appointment, but sometimes they don't, so that's the first step. Our records technician will grab them from the waiting room and take photos and x-rays. The records techs have about an eight-minute window to take the full records. Then, the TC will go over their health history and other important things on the paperwork while the records are being printed. Then, we ask the doctor to come in, and they typically have a two-minute window in the room, so they're in and out pretty quickly. It's the TC doing a lot of talking after that, like going over fees and commitments."

So let's discuss this formula and some of the best practices you can implement to make it happen for your practice.

First, commit to making the 60-minute consultation a thing of the past. Make sure your entire team has bought in to this concept. If they're not willing to join you in this exciting process, that's okay—it's their choice. But you absolutely need the right people on your team if you want to grow.

Next, realize that it is not the length of the appointment that creates patient satisfaction. A long, inefficient appointment with staff that would rather be at home binge-watching a show is a real turn off. No amount of doctor time with nice lengthy explanations can make up for poor customer service. Everyone on your team must be committed to wowing your patients with efficiency, competence, and kindness. Most of all, the patients will appreciate the convenience of not having to take more time off work or school.

Now let's delve into the details so you can free up time for you and your team to grow!

## 8-Minute Records

Humans find the concept of change difficult. It's hard to wrap your head around doing things differently than you're used to. That's why innovators often practice changing up the smallest things like the order in which they floss their teeth or the route they take to the office. Little practices like this can get you more accepting to a change in perspective.

I'm sure if you bring this up with your records techs right now, they'll give you all sorts of reasons why it's going to be a problem like, "It takes me this long to take x-rays and photos and make sure they turn out right. Or I like to take my time to make sure the patient knows what I'm doing and is comfortable with everything. Or I need to make sure everything is set up in this particular way and I can't do it any faster." This is normal.

To open them up to the concept of a faster way, find an office where the techs are doing 8-minute records and ask if your staff can observe the process. Maybe you can arrange a call with their records tech so they can give your techs tips on how they could speed up their process. There are also in-office courses that teach office procedures that can be really helpful in changing your whole office's mindset really fast.

Make time to train on the process. Practice with each other and time the process from start to finish. Keep running through it until you can perform all the x-rays and photos in eight minutes or less. Doing it with another team member gives you the freedom to make mistakes and ask questions. It's okay if this takes a little time to perfect. Celebrate the improvements your team makes and keep practicing.

Kasey explains what Dr. Fishbein did to help his record techs eventually reach their goal time:

*"Dr. Fishbein would secretly time our record techs and praise them whenever they got quicker. It would get better and better every time he did it, and now they're all at 8 minutes. But now they're so motivated, they even want to beat that time! They know they have another patient coming in every 15 minutes, so they want to be quick."*

Encourage them to try to beat their best time each week and set a bonus for every time they do.

## 2-Minute Doctor Consultation

Let's take a moment to think about the real outcome that we are anticipating from this free consultation. As a doctor, it's common place to think it's time to discuss the clinical presentation of the patient's case and show them what's going on in their mouth from a medical standpoint. While this makes sense, it does not really serve the purpose of convincing the person to start treatment. In order for you to put your clinical skills to work and transform this person's life, they must first agree to the treatment plan and fees. We don't want too many details to affect the prospective patient's ability to make a decision on starting treatment at your practice.

There is a balance between sharing medical information with the patient and reassuring them that the process is straightforward and easy. In fact, data proves that information overload will in fact cause the prospective patient to have analysis paralysis. "Is this going to hurt... it sounds painful! OMG, what is class 2... that sounds serious. Wow, what if I have to have surgery to correct this? Teeth pulled?! OUCH!! I am not really sure what he is talking about... I might just get a second opinion." While some medical details are valid and may need to be communicated, a TC will keep these explanations very simple and focus on keeping the patient at ease.

Simply put, the more they are told, the more questions that come up. They'll have to talk to their spouse, their friends, their family, and worst of all, another orthodontist. If the other office puts them at ease, reassures them that it's no problem, and in fact, it's so simple that they can get started today, guess what? You spent the marketing dollars, did all the work, got them primed and ready to take care of the problem, and the other doctor got the $5000-$7000.

So what is the purpose of the consultation from a purely operational point of view? It's to reassure the patient that they are in the right place, with kind people who care about them, and who have the competence to change the mess in their mouth into the smile they want.

As the doctor, all you need to do is review the x-rays and photos the records technicians provided and relay the treatment plan to the patient in layman's terms. They know their teeth need work, what are you going to do to fix it? Braces? Invisalign? Headgear? How long will it take? 6 months, 12 months, 24 months? This really shouldn't take more than 2 minutes to do. Introduce yourself, briefly explain the treatment plan, re-direct their attention to the TC for the fee presentation, and say your farewells until next time. That's it. This is your TC's time to shine—you're only there to meet them and inspire confidence.

Obviously, there will be times that may take longer, but for the most part those are pretty few and far between. The point here is that there is a big opportunity in optimizing the process to be as efficient as possible.

Kasey has seen how long doctor consults can backfire, so she understands the importance of keeping it short and sweet:

> "I think when the doctor spends 20 minutes in the exam room going super in-depth about the science of orthodontics with

*the patient, they end up taking all this information in, and they feel like it's a big deal and it's something they need to go home and digest. And that's not what we want. So we try to keep every part of the process extremely simple, including the doctor's portion of the exam. I think that helps a lot with eliminating objections."*

Some doctors are now reviewing the records and giving the findings and recommendation to the TC to relay to the patient. They call this a TC Empowerment Consultation. The TC provides the treatment recommendations to the patient on the doctor's behalf and then proceeds to discuss the finances. You may be thinking that this would decrease the conversion rate because there is no connection with the doctor at all during the first visit. Would you believe that these offices actually found their conversion rate increased?

My theory is that most orthodontists are much more in their element when they are chairside with patients. Meeting new people and navigating the different emotions and objections that come up is not usually their thing. The patient is inspired by the confidence of the TC, their experience at the clinic has been top-notch so far, therefore it just makes sense that the orthodontist will be on par with their team.

Listen to Dr. Ben Fishbein talk about the implementation of doctorless consults in his office.

If you feel you won't have the time to do the comprehensive examination and treatment planning that the patient needs to receive a high standard of care, consider this. Once the patient has committed to the process and put their financial concerns behind them, you can focus completely on the examination and treatment plan knowing that your time has already been paid for. You will have a couple of years to get to know that patient and build a rapport. It doesn't have to take place during a time-sensitive exam that your TC is more than capable of handling on their own. Put your trust in them; they know what to do to get your patients in the chair!

## 5-Minute Fee Presentation

At the end of the day, the only reason that the patient has taken you up on the offer for a free consultation is to find out the cost of straightening their teeth. The fee presentation is the most important part of the consultation for conversion. They already know that their teeth are crooked since they see them every day. People are always interested to learn about procedures that will improve the way they look, but their guards go up when it comes to discussing the actual cost. Fees will always be the number one objection to starting.

A $5000-$7000 decision for most people is outside of their comfort zone, however, if their crooked teeth are affecting their confidence, moving forward with treatment is the best decision they can make. It is your duty to provide them with the means to say 'yes' by making treatment financially feasible for them, without it impacting their day-to-day living or breaking the bank.

We want to make sure we can eliminate this objection from the get-go, so any discussion about fees should be presented early on in the discourse with the patient. It should begin as soon as your scheduling coordinators have their first conversation during the new patient phone call. While it would be impossible to give an exact cost to patients at this point, the scheduling coordinator should be able to pre-frame pricing by presenting what the average breakdown is.

Here's an example of what your scheduling coordinators could say to pre-frame pricing:

- *We do need to see you for an exam, which is free of charge, to be able to give you an accurate fee and treatment plan, only because the fee depends on how long the doctor says you will need to be in treatment. Some people are in treatment for 12 months, some for over 24 months. BUT what I CAN tell you is that we do have super affordable payment plans for everyone, all in-house, at 0% interest to you, no credit checks, and most people can start treatment for as little as $X down and monthly payments as low as $X per month. Could that possibly work for you?"*

If your scheduling coordinators are pre-framing pricing like this in the initial phone call, it will ensure that your patients are kept informed and will eliminate any surprises or objections during the consultation with the TC. Teamwork is essential, so this is a crucial first step.

TCs should also avoid using the "big number" and instead lead with one payment plan that includes a low down payment, and a monthly fee structure. This is the best way to ease people's anxieties regarding fees. It has to be presented in the simplest way possible to decrease the patient's chance of needing to "think about it." Through trial and error, our most successful clients have found that the fee presentation shouldn't take longer than five minutes, and must include only one option.

Kasey has tried numerous approaches over the years as a TC, but she feels pretty confident with Dr. Fishbein's current fee presentation method now:

"Our fee presentation is pretty simple, so it takes five minutes every time, no matter what. We only give them one *fee option because we don't want them to be confused by so many options. The main obstacle will always be fees, so we have focused so much on simplifying the estimate process over the years, and it's very streamlined now. We do the same thing every single time. This typically helps eliminate any questions from the patient. We don't give any other options, so there's really nothing to be overwhelmed by, which means they won't have to go home and talk to their spouse about it.*"

Okay, so what is the option? How do I make the presentation five minutes? How can it be presented simply? We will answer these questions in full detail in the following chapter.

## Virtual Consultations

As horrible as the pandemic was over the last few years, it did help the world see that it's possible to do many things from the comfort and protection of your own home, like work, school, and even appointments! Many practices have been able to offer virtual consultations during the pandemic, and they have been so successful that a lot of practices are making them a permanent thing. Offering a virtual consultation to patients is a convenient service that can help them maximize their time, so they don't have to leave work or school (or even their home) for multiple appointments.

The process of the virtual appointment is pretty straightforward: the patient submits information and photos of their teeth from different angles to the office, and the office sends back the treatment plan and the financial option. If they are interested in starting treatment upon receiving that information, they will then schedule their in-office consultation and start on the same day. That's all that's involved! Quick, efficient, and convenient.

Stacey Bagwell, the Treatment Coordinator from Weldman Orthodontics, and her team decided to implement virtual consultations in their practice in 2019. Here's what she had to say about its success:

> "Our virtual consults is an evolving process. It was a DIY when we first decided to do it, but then we started using SmileSnap, which helped us streamline our work more efficiently. SmileSnap is integrated within our Slack messaging system, so any updates we receive from patients are automatically populated in the Slack channel. The patient just has to submit their photos to us using this channel, and from there, the doctor can review them and provide a customized treatment plan with a quote. If the patient agrees to move forward with treatment, we'll get them in the office and take more records on their start date."

Stacey even reveals how the virtual consultations have doubled the practice's adult conversion rate:

> "This process has worked so well for us that we've decided to make it permanent. Working professionals prefer it this way because it gets things moving quickly without booking time off from work. And our close rate is pretty good, as 50% of them are pre-qualified and are most likely to start treatment the same day they come in for their in-office consultation. Our adult conversion rate actually doubled since we began to offer virtual consultations. We are now thinking of new ways to make it even better to maximize the patient experience."

If you don't use SmileSnap or Rhinogram, you can still do this by using our system, PracticeBeacon (PB). PB will follow up with the patient and prompt a call with the office. If the patient submitted photos, they can expect a free quote and treatment plan later that day via the PB chat. The scheduling coordinator will then schedule the person to come in for the consult and same-day start. The remaining elements can occur when the prospect comes into the office.

Ultimately, the virtual consultation is a quick way to pre-qualify patients and determine those most likely to start treatment. It will help your practice save time and allow your team to consult with patients who are interested in moving forward. This can only be achieved if it is pre-framed, like everything else, in the initial phone call with your scheduling coordinators. Virtual consultations are especially helpful if the patient can't get scheduled for an in-office consultation within 72 hours.

Here's how your scheduling coordinators can present this option to patients, either by phone call or text message:

If calling the patient:

**Option 1:**
- *...You will love our virtual process! I will text/email you some easy instructions to begin. You simply answer a few questions, submit a few photos of your teeth, and we will be back in touch with all of the information you need to get started with your treatment, including fees.*

**Option 2:**
- *Our next available appointment is [date], but we can go ahead and get the process started today!! We are going to text you some simple instructions—all you have to do is answer a few questions and submit a few photos of your teeth. We will get back to you later today with a free quote and our treatment plan, and our Treatment Coordinator can call to review the quote and next steps. How's that sound?!*

*Please note: Both of these options would come after establishing the appointment and would need to be scheduled past three days from the time of the call.

**Follow-up text, after the call with the patient:**

- *Hi [first name], we're so excited to help you with your orthodontic needs. Here are the angles of your teeth you need to take photos of to get started. Once I receive your photos, we will be in touch with the quote and treatment plan within an hour! P.S. I may have a few questions based on your photos!*

*You can also use this for Observation, Recall, Aligner Checks, and Retainer Patients!

If texting the parent of a patient:

- *Hi [first name], [patient name] is due for a follow-up visit with Dr.[name]. Can you text us these photo angles so we can evaluate treatment virtually and see if an in-person visit is needed? If everything looks good, then we can save you a trip!*

If you've never heard of a virtual consultation, start thinking about implementing it in your practice ASAP. This will not only make the in-office consultations easier for your TC, but it will guarantee more serious candidates who are ready to start treatment when they walk through your doors.

## Are You Ready to Say Goodbye to the 60-Minute Consultation?

It's entirely possible to get your new patient consultation down to 30 minutes (or even shorter) with the 8-minute records, 2-5-minute doctor consultations, and 5-minute fee presentation formula. Dozens of the practices I work with are making great strides to transition their teams to this format.

Mary Scott, the Treatment Coordinator at AllSmiles Orthodontics, tells us how her team has made an effort to get the consultation time down to 30 minutes and the benefits it has caused:

> "We used to have people come in for an exam, come back a few days later for all their records, and then come back two weeks later for the doctor to present the treatment plan. So it used to be a month-long process. We tried to shorten it, and we were a bit successful, but it's nothing like it is now. Getting everything done all within 30 minutes and having the patient able to start that same day has really helped so many families. And that's what HIP helped us learn: we were always looking at it from our perspective and not the patient's perspective. It has helped us realize that it's not always what is best for us but what is best for the patient."

Mary continues:

> "I started working with this newly graduated doctor at our office a while back. When he first began doing consultations, he wanted to take his time going over records. He wouldn't even come into the exam without planning everything out. And I think many doctors want to do that so they can be completely thorough with the patient during the exam. With the help of HIP, the doctors realize that they don't have to treatment plan the whole thing: they just have to deliver what we know we can do and not get into all the details. It's helped us not overwhelm the families with the information they don't need. The doctors have even learned how to change their dialogue and delivery to quickly get in and out to keep that exam short and sweet. Then, onto the next all over again."

## Slow and Steady Wins the Race

Don't expect to read about this today and have it all working in your office tomorrow. Every practice featured in this book who took the time and effort to bring the consultation time down from 60 minutes to 30 minutes did so by first committing to the process of change. They got their team on board, set targets, and remained consistent in training and practice. If you follow the steps I've laid out for you, this can happen in your office and make all the difference in your practice growth.

In the next chapter, we'll dive deep into one of the most important strategies your TC will need to know to succeed: The 5-Minute Fee Presentation that will up your conversion rate to between 75 and 80%.

# CHAPTER 4
# Employing Fee and Pricing Strategies

*"Every sale has five basic obstacles: no need, no money, no hurry, no desire, no trust."*

*– Zig Ziglar*

Picture this: you're watching TV when a car commercial comes on. It's a beautiful, new luxury sports car driving down the Pacific Coast Highway during a picturesque golden California sunset. You think to yourself: You know what, it's time for me to buy a sports car. I want to be coasting in it down the highway, too! I work hard—I deserve it. Then, suddenly, the price comes up: "$80,000—it could be yours today!" Mhm, no, it can't. And so you turn off the TV and accept your mediocre sedan as "good enough" for now.

This doesn't happen and people buy cars that are more expensive than their household income can support every day because the car company knows you want that luxury sports car. They're not going to scare you away with the car's huge price tag. Instead, they tell you that the car can be yours, "starting at $x/month, with 0% down and x% interest rate." They know how to get people to the dealership because once they sit in the car, it's game over. They're definitely not paying $80,000 out of pocket today, unless they're insanely rich and have that kind of disposable income, but they will drive it off the lot today if they can manage the monthly payments.

49

The same goes for orthodontic treatment. Many of your patients may have a child that needs orthodontic treatment or in some cases, multiple children. Other patients may be students working part-time to save up for the treatment or adults working full-time who can use their insurance to cover a portion of the cost. For most people, a treatment that costs over $5000 is too much money to dish out, so your TC must be able to present fees to patients without causing their alarm bells to ring. Here's how your TC can do this the right way.

## Avoid Saying the "Big Number" Out Loud

Just as with all the procedures we've discussed so far, the set up for this starts with your scheduling coordinators. Since they're the first to engage with prospective patients, they are the ones who need to pre-frame treatment costs. However, everyone in the office needs to be aware of how pricing is discussed to ensure that they're all on the same page and presenting a unified front.

The scheduling coordinators are the first ones that should be avoiding that big number and providing the prospective patient with an average price breakdown, including the down payment and monthly fee. This is absolutely crucial for your TC. They won't be able to avoid the big number completely as patients do need to know the overall cost of treatment, but there are still good ways to do this without activating their anxieties and getting their objections to kick in. It's as simple as just pointing to the number instead of saying it. I'll show you how you can put this into practice later in the chapter.

## Offer One Pricing Option

We are fortunate enough to live in a world with many options available to us. Do I want Mexican or Italian for lunch? Do I want to buy this cheaper jacket from the department store or the-one-of-a-kind piece from that boutique? Should I spend my birthday money on clothes or put it in my savings account? It's great to have options, but if you're not an impulsive risk-taker, options usually come with the need to make a decision, and making the right decision usually requires time. As a practice trying to take on more patients, giving numerous options isn't exactly the best method to attain growth. When you offer multiple pricing or payment options to a patient, you force them to make more decisions which can cause them to hesitate. And then you'll hear:

- *I need to talk to my husband/wife/partner about this.*
- *I need to think about it.*
- *I'm not sure right now. Can I get back to you?*

So, you need to make it as easy as possible for them to say 'yes.' How? You need to instruct your TC to lead by giving patients one simple and easy-to-understand payment option, where the price is digestible and reasonable to commit to. After working with hundreds of practices on this, we've realized that the best structure is this: **A down payment of $300 or less, plus monthly payments of $200 or less.**

Few people feel the need to go home and think it over at these prices. If the patient would like to put down more to lower their monthly fee, then let them be the ones to suggest it.

Kasey from Fishbein explains how this works:

"*The patient shouldn't have to decide between the four options I've suggested. We used to do that, and everyone needed to think it over. Now, we always lead with that*

51

*payment plan of $300 down, and it has to be less than $200 per month. That's our TCs rule for financing, and that typically eliminates any questions from the patient. If the patient wants to put down more or pay in full, we will discuss it. However, we will never lead with that. They can make their suggestions afterward, and we will ultimately do whatever they feel comfortable with.*"

If you get your TC to do this every time with every patient, you will see how quickly your conversion rates rise.

## Always Mention Coverage, Discounts, and Promotions

People love getting a good deal so what better way to get someone on board with treatment than by telling them how much money they get to save! When your TC presents the treatment plan to patients, they should always include the amount covered by their insurance and any promotions and discounts currently taking place in your office before they provide the payment structure. This way, when they present the final fees, they can give the price breakdown with the savings already factored in, and assure them that they're getting the lowest rate possible.

For example, if their insurance covers $1000 and your practice is offering $500 off treatment for June, make sure your TC factors that in before they crunch the numbers. It will lower their overall fee and boost their confidence in knowing they're getting a sweet deal.

## Be Flexible

If your TC offers this payment plan and the patient is still hesitant to start, they have to be empathetic and offer some flexibility. As a practice that values its patients, you want to be able to do everything in your power to keep the patient happy and do what you can to accommodate them. If they're hesitant about the down payment, your TC can offer to split it in half where they pay $150 today and the other $150 in two weeks. This can make a big difference to a person's cashflow when they get paid every two weeks. If they struggle with the $200 monthly fee, expand their payment plan beyond their treatment deadline by a few months to achieve a lower monthly rate. [Hear Madison's fee presentation by scanning the QR code below.] They'll still be coming into the office for their retainer checks over the next 6 months after treatment is completed, so it's easy to pitch extended treatment plans beyond 24 months.

## The Fee Presentation

This is where all of the magic happens and it shouldn't take longer than 5 minutes. If you're using the strategies listed above, you will have no problem making this happen. But let's tie it all together so you can see how it actually looks. And no, you don't need an overhead projector or iPad showcasing a detailed PowerPoint presentation to do this successfully. You really only need a piece of paper outlining their financial agreement and a pen for them to sign.

Here's what HIP's Orthodontic Financial Agreement looks like:

## Orthodontic Financial Agreement

Date: _____ Start Date: _____
Responsible Party: _____ Phone Number: _____
Patient: _____ Email: _____
_____ Full Treatment _____ Phase I _____ Phase II _____ ETT
_____ Limited Treatment _____ Invisalign _____ Incognito
  1. Professional Fee                         $ _____

  2. Less Applicable Courtesy _____ % _____     $ _____

  3. Less Estimated Insurance          $ _____

  4. Estimated Responsible Party Portion   $ _____

  5. Less Initial Payment [Due_____]    $ _____

  6. Unpaid Balance                    $ _____

Unpaid balance [#6] above is payable to _____ in _____
_____ monthly installments of $ _____ each, and one
installment of the remaining balance. The first initial
payment is payable on _____ and subsequent installments
on the same day of each consecutive month until paid in
full. A $10 late fee will be charged on all accounts that
are 10 days past due.

_____    _____    _____
Signature           Witness           Date

*I understand that this amount is an estimate only and
that I am personally responsible for any balance not
paid by insurance.

If your TC presents this to their patients, it should already
be filled out. Everything should be outlined, including the
total treatment cost, insurance coverage, promotions, down
payment, and monthly fee structure. All they have to do at
the end of the presentation is sign and date it.

Here's how this looks in practice:

- *Okay, [patient's name], this is your total treatment fee...*
  *Point to the number [$5800] but don't say it out loud*

- *Here's some really good news, [patient's name], you've got awesome insurance that will cover $2000 of your treatment fee, which is amazing. That leaves you with $3800. You can take care of that however you want, but just as a starting place to make it easy and convenient for you, if you put down $300 today, your monthly payment will be $179/month over the next 24 months. Is that something that might possibly work for you?*
  *Then, stop talking!*
  *9/10 times, they will say that works for them*

- *Okay, great. How do you want to take care of the $300 down payment today? Amex,Visa, or...?*

## The Top 1% Orthodontic Clinics Are Doing It and So Can You!

Your new patients really want to start treatment. It's up to your TC to help them get past the common obstacles that stand in their way. Following these pricing strategies exemplified by the nation's fastest-growing orthodontic practices will help you get more patients starting treatment as soon as today. In the next chapter, we will go into detail about how you can make that close stick with the same-day start.

# CHAPTER 5

# Positioning the Same-Day Start

*"One day or day one. You decide."*

— Paulo Coelho

Throughout this book, we have been talking about how some offices are having great success with getting patients to begin treatment on the same day as they have their free consultation. For many offices, it can take several weeks between the initial consultation and starting treatment. You may be wondering why it is so important to get the patient in the chair so quickly. The answer is human nature.

In any B2C business, the hardest part of the sales process is getting people to overcome their inertia and take action. All of your team's efforts in marketing, follow up, and scheduling to get that lead to the new patient consultation is to give your TC that one opportunity to convert them into a start. Once the orthodontist has given their recommendations for treatment, there is a brief window where they are primed and ready to commit to the lengthy and expensive process. You need to make your move, get that commitment, and make it stick. The way to do this is by getting a credit card on file, taking the down payment, and getting the braces on their teeth. This way, all the financial uncertainty is behind them and they have taken the leap. There's no turning back. If they do, they've paid to get the braces on and they must make an effort to reverse the decision they made.

You might think that scheduling them to come back for their treatment plan or start is enough of a commitment but as soon as they leave your office, the doubts creep in and they begin talking themselves out of the process. Even if they have given you a credit card or made a payment, if they have not received any service beyond the free consultation, they can get a refund.

Worst of all, they have your pricing and can do some comparison shopping. Since your TC is not there to explain the value of your treatment plan, a TC from another office who is skilled in conversion could get them to start treatment even if their prices are higher. You and your team did all the work getting them motivated to straighten their teeth; the other office simply stepped in, got them started, and added the $5000-$7000 to their production.

They showed up to your office for a reason. Nobody takes a day off to go to an orthodontist's office simply to pass the time unless they are considering investing in braces. They value their time as much, if not more, than their money. If they've chosen to come to your office, they've already decided that they want to start treatment. When? Probably whenever is most convenient for them. If they're here now, it saves taking more time off and another trip. That's pretty convenient. However, they won't know that a same-day start is an option unless they are told. This chapter will discuss the strategies your TC and the rest of your team can use to identify and eliminate objections that keep your patients from confidently and willingly saying 'yes' to starting treatment that same day.

## It All Starts with Your Scheduling Coordinators

Getting a 'yes' to a same-day start begins at the very first contact with the lead, so pre-framing the same-day start is the key to success. It is critical that your scheduling coordinators tell the lead about the low down payment and monthly fee structure, as well as the opportunity to same-day start. Once they've gathered all the necessary information from the patient and the consultation is set, here's how to close the conversation:

- *It was great speaking with you today, [patient's name]. Did you have any other questions for us?*

- *Ok, awesome! When you come in, you will meet with one of our awesome Treatment Coordinators, [TC name], take some photos and x-rays, and the doctor will do an exam. The consultation is free of charge to you. Please allow about one hour for your appointment. If the doctor does think that you're ready for treatment, we can actually go ahead and get your treatment started that same day so that you do not have to come back for another appointment, if that might be convenient for you?*

- *Thank you so much for calling, and we look forward to seeing you at your appointment!*

Making this pre-framing a mandatory part of the scheduling procedure sets your TC up for success. We don't want the patient to be surprised by the option to same-day start. If they are not pre-framed, we don't know what they are they're thinking. They won't necessarily have allowed time for the start or be ready to commit to a payment plan. Simply making sure that your scheduling coordinators are well versed with this script and use it to schedule every new patient consultation will increase your conversion rate.

Vanessa from Knecht Orthodontics always makes sure her scheduling coordinators are aware of how this helps when she's trying to close a sale:

> "I always tell our scheduling coordinators, 'Make sure it's being pre-framed in the new patient phone call!' I say this because it can eliminate objections during the consultation. Most patients ask if they can start that same day because our scheduling coordinator told them that it's an option during their first call. So I don't even have to bring it up sometimes because they're suggesting it! It's great. People love its convenience because the last thing they want to do is book more time off work to come here."

Potential patients may have waited weeks, months, or years to reach out to your office. They may have even heard great things about your practice from their referring dentist. When they finally decide to contact your office, they have already made up their minds that they need to invest in braces and they want results now. By following our "Speed to Lead" strategy, more pre-framed leads will get booked for consultations and your TC's conversion rate will go up, adding more to production every month.

We covered "Speed to Lead" in detail in *Front Desk Secrets*, but for a quick review, it means your scheduling coordinators respond to leads within 5 minutes of contact, book free consultations within 72 hours, and schedule virtual exams for those who can't make it within that time frame. If this becomes standard practice for your office, your team will wow new patients with their customer service and efficiency and instill confidence that the orthodontic treatment you provide is top-notch. This will build a connection with them, making it easier for your TC to get them on board.

Mary from AllSmiles quickly saw how impactful the same-day start was, but also how it involved a team effort to be effective:

> "We saw how well Fishbein was doing with the same-day starts, so we followed their lead. We noticed how they introduced the notion of a same-day start in the introductory phone call to the patient, which would help them plant the seed. It then becomes a layering process throughout. We've realized that if we layer it correctly, things seamlessly flow—people are ready to accept the treatment and start the same day. It's amazing, but it's a team effort. I actually just had a patient who wasn't sure about the same-day start. Still, I kept an understanding tone and said, "I totally understand; we just suggested it only if it's convenient for you and your family." By the end of the conversation, she said, "Well, if my son wants to start that day, then sure, I suppose we can." I guess I got her to lower her guard a bit. I love how all these pieces keep coming together, and we're getting the process all refined."

## Is the Same-Day Start Possible for Every Practice?

It can be overwhelming to think of all the steps that your team will have to take to get new patients to start on the same day. You definitely can't read this book over the weekend and expect to change things on Monday. It would be way too overwhelming for your team. The first step is to make sure you have the right people and processes in place. If you are committed to growing your practice and follow the steps I've shared so far in the Orthodontic Practice Growth Series, you will be able to make this a reality in your office.

Fishbein Orthodontics hasn't always offered same-day starts, but they've only seen positive results since implemented. Here's what Kasey has to say about it:

> "When I first started, same-day starts were a foreign concept for our office—we didn't do many of them. We expect at least ten same-day starts per location per day now. Our team and clinics know to expect it, and it's definitely a TC mindset. We're making it convenient for our patients by saving them time. But you need to have the right people to make it happen smoothly. Everyone needs to have a role so we can make that 30-minute exam and have everything taking place within that move smoothly and efficiently."

## What if We Do Invisalign?

It's understandable how getting the process of braces started can make the sale stick. The braces literally get bonded to their teeth. It takes effort to undo. So how can we do a same-day start with Invisalign? With iTero scanning, why would they pay you before they get their first tray? Where's the urgency to make a financial commitment?

The TC creates a sense of urgency by explaining that there is a two to four-week turnaround from the time the office submits the treatment plan to when the lab team at Invisalign makes and delivers the trays. Getting the patient scanned during the consultation saves them the hassle of another trip back to the office, which means they can be fitted for their first tray the next time they come in.

Offering to split the down payment can come in handy, too. The TC can offer to take half the down payment after the fee presentation and do the iTero scan the same day. The second half of the down payment is charged when they come back for the Inv delivery.

# But What If Patients Don't Want a Same-Day Start?

The national conversion rate on orthodontic exams is just over 50%, which means that something stops nearly half of patients from starting a treatment they really want. Unfortunately, this opens up the opportunity to start with a competitor or DIYer that has a better sales process. Most of the time, they have objections: either they're overwhelmed by fees, uncertain about timing and scheduling for themselves or their children, or they're unsatisfied with your service. In order to eliminate these objections and get them started, let's take a moment to understand why they are saying 'no.'

In order for a person to commit to a lengthy process involving a large sum of money, the following four factors must be part of their decision-making process:

1. Do they have the **time** to follow through with the process and get results?
2. Do they have an **understanding** of how the process works?
3. Do they have the **authority** to make the decision?
4. Do they have the **money** to pay for it?

Here's how your TC can address all four factors when presenting the fees.

- *Okay, great. Now that you've heard from the doctor, there are a few things we need to discuss to make sure that you can commit to the treatment plan so that you can get the smile that you want!*
- **Time:** *Will you be able to come back every 6 weeks for check-ins? Is that something you can commit to?*
- **Understanding:** *Can you promise me you will [wear your aligners or rubber bands; eat the right foods; come in to fix a broken wire ASAP]? Can you do that for me?*

- **Authority:** *My awesome scheduling coordinator, [name], said that you would be taking care of the treatment cost. Is that still the case, or is there anybody else that might be involved in the financial decision?*

- **Money:** *Okay, great. If that all sounds good, this is where we would go over the financial agreement, if that feels appropriate to you?*

Since the goal of the TC role is to ensure that patient obstacles are identified and eliminated, asking the right questions and offering solutions to ease concerns is paramount. It doesn't take long to do this: their answers to the four simple questions above gauge how serious the patient is about committing to treatment. If they are hesitant to answer one of the questions, there might be objections to address. Ask them specifically what is getting in the way of them being able to start treatment.

If it is an issue of **time**, it may just require reassurance that scheduling will not be an issue for them. For example, if their concern is taking time off work or school and you offer evening appointments, you could encourage them to reserve all their appointments in advance to make sure they always know they have a spot that fits in their schedule.

If they appear to have trouble **understanding** the treatment plan or fees, you may need to get the doctor to come back to answer any questions they may have about the process. If they are having issues with the fees, it may be that you need to address the next two factors.

It could be that they do not feel they have the **authority** to make such a big expenditure without consulting their spouse. For example, if they need to run it by their husband or wife before saying 'yes,' you can simply say:

- *I totally understand, [patient's name]. I will leave the room, close the door, and give you the privacy to give him/her a call. Just open the door whenever you're finished and take all the time you need.*

After speaking with numerous TCs for research for this book, these patients take that option 90% of the time. They give their spouse/partner a call in the room, and it usually gets sorted out, and the same-day start takes place. Because let's face it, no one likes to have a private conversation about money with the salesperson in the room staring at them. That will only make them more uncomfortable, causing their guard to go up even higher, followed by an awkward, "No, it's okay. I will speak to them in private when I get home."

Mary from AllSmiles uses this strategy to get her patients to say 'yes' comfortably:

> "If we go over the financial agreement and they still want to discuss the fees with their spouse, we will say something like, "I understand; this is a big decision. We can step out of the room for a minute if you want to give them a call or FaceTime, and we can answer any questions you both have. Most of the time, they actually will call their spouse and take care of it then and there. They usually give the go-ahead, and we end up being able to start that day."

From the previous chapter, you already know that **money** and fees are the number one patient objection to starting treatment. If your TC follows the advice in Chapter 4 by offering one pricing option, a deposit and monthly payment structure, and flexibility in extended payments, more often than not, they will not have an objection to the fees.

## What If the Patient is Still Unsure?

What if you've followed all these steps and despite your best efforts, the patient is still hesitant to start? In this case, there's probably another objection to address. If the patient turns down your offer to call their spouse/partner privately in the room, other factors may be at play. Maybe they can't afford to pay the $300 down payment right now? Perhaps they know their spouse/partner will automatically turn down treatment because the upfront costs are too expensive? Whatever the reason is, it's valid. Families have enormous expenses to take care of—life is not cheap. I understand, having a family myself.

If this happens, there are a few things your TC can do to help move the process along, however, before trying to use other tactics, your TC must always lead with empathy. This is not the time to be judgemental or unkind. Discussing finances is a touchy subject for many people, so they should always keep that in mind as the financial discussion continues. Saying things like, "I understand how you feel," or "I get it's difficult committing to this right now," can be helpful to show people that you hear them and care.

Mary from AllSmiles always comes from a place of empathy when having these financial conversations with patients, and it's because of her own experiences as a mother:

> "I try not to be so cavalier with people's money. I try to put myself in my patient's position and understand how it's tough for some people regarding money and finances. $7000 for braces is a lot of money. I remember when my daughter needed help with her reading, so we got her in this extended reading program, and it was around $5000. And when they presented the fees, they didn't have options for a low down payment. They had a standard monthly fee with interest, and I remember feeling overwhelmed by the price and how she was presenting it to me. So I try to empathize

*with patients and do my best to work out a plan that can help them."*

Here are some strategies that your TC can consider to help patients get on board:

1. **Split the down payment:** Your TC can help patients with their down payment by splitting it in half. If the down payment is $300, they can pay $150 today and the other $150 in two weeks. Since most people get paid biweekly, it can be advantageous to split the cost, so they aren't spending a chunk of their paycheck this week on treatment costs. Many patients take advantage of this, especially those uncomfortable with the upfront costs. Therefore, if they were feeling iffy about calling their spouse/partner before, suggest this and ask them to make the call to share this new information. 95% of the time, they'll move forward with a same-day start.

2. **Match the down payment:** Right now, we're seeing the "down payment match" promotion work wonders at industry-leading practices. You can tell the patient that during this month, patients who start care right away get the added benefit of the clinic matching their $300 down payment. Fishbein Orthodontics runs this promotion a few months a year. In terms of this promotion, Kasey says, "Even if they felt like they didn't have the money, they're finding a way to get the money." It's quite an incentive because if they go home to think about it, they won't get the deal. If this is not something that is financially feasible for your practice, consider the next point.

3. **Offer cool gifts:** Smaller take-home gifts such as Gobi toothbrushes, Propel VPro5 mouthpieces, or even Zoom whitening kits for patients who start right away can be enough to tip them over the edge.

But despite all efforts, that patient still may not start. Mary understands that there comes a point when you have to stop and encourage the patient to come back when they're ready:

> "You can offer all that, but you can only do so much. One patient I recently saw was struggling with the fees I was presenting. I offered to divide her down payment into two payments, but she still couldn't do it. She had five kids and just couldn't add another bill at this time. So you have to understand that it's hard for people to commit sometimes. You have to do your best to accommodate, but ultimately know when to stop pushing and let them know you'll be there for them when they are ready."

Your TC must understand that they can't push, persuade, or manipulate people to make a decision they simply cannot make. While they should always do their best to get treatment started, if the patient can't begin that same day, they need to be aware that your practice will always be there for them. It's important for your clinic to stay top of mind because, when their circumstances change, and they're ready to move forward with treatment, you want to make sure they come to your office rather than jumping on another clinic's special introductory offer. To stay on your patient's radar, it's imperative that your TC has the proper tracking and follow up system, which is the topic of the next chapter.

Your TC shouldn't have to convince new patients to start treatment. They simply need to show them that their fears are unnecessary; that they can get their desired results without putting undue financial pressure on their families or disrupting their lifestyle. By making the consultation experience as straightforward as possible and having empathy for the patient's wants, fears, and objections, the TC can make it easy for them to move forward with the same-day start. You'll find that new patients are saying 'yes' much more than ever, and they're excited to start treatment and are thrilled with their results.

CHAPTER **6**

# Tracking and Following-Up with Pending Patients

*"Follow up and follow through until the task is completed, the prize won."*

— Brian Tracy

The end goal of every new patient consultation is to hear the word 'yes.' We want them to agree to the fees, make a down payment, and get in the chair to start treatment. If they can't start the same day, we want them scheduled to come back for their start. If neither of these two options happen, their file moves to pending and in a lot of offices, that's the end of story.

Your team is committed to helping patients to do what's best for them, so it can be a real blow to hear the word 'no.' Once you implement the processes in this book, that should happen a lot less. In fact, you should see that this only happens less than 25% of the time. However, no matter how good your team gets with these systems, about one out of every four new patients will not be ready to move forward with treatment.

When a potential patient leaves your office without saying 'yes,' the chances of them ever starting care in your office drop dramatically. That chance drops to almost zero if your TC gives up on them. That's why having well-defined follow-up practices for pending patients is crucial. This chapter outlines how your TC can effectively track and follow up with pending patients to turn that 'maybe' into 'yes'!

## Don't Give Up on Them!

It can be demoralizing to put your whole heart into something and not get the results you were hoping for, but it's important to keep the right attitude. These people aren't all solid 'nos.' You just have to see them as, "not right nows." All they need is someone caring to check in with them on a regular basis to see whether they are ready to start. The magic is in the follow up.

Tracking and follow up can be time-consuming and it's the first thing to fall through the cracks when the days get busy. But you can make it easy. It starts with getting your team in the right mindset around pending patients, and having systems to make sure follow-up happens every day.

It should be exciting to look at your list of pendings and see how much money is sitting there waiting to be tapped. These are all people who self-identified, saying, "I really want a better smile." They wanted it badly enough to book an appointment and show up for a consultation. Maybe today the timing is right for them to say 'yes'!

TCs have a million things to do every day, just to take care of the new patient consultations coming in. It's natural to prioritize them because they're potential 'yeses,' but dropping the people in the 'maybe' category is leaving a lot of money on the table. With the right systems for tracking and follow up, your office can get a lot of these people to start, and best of all, the hard work has already been done.

Encourage your TC to follow up with pending patients every

week for at least a month. They're not being a bother. They're helping these people to stay focused on the smile they always dreamed of. When your TC follows up, they're just offering assistance by removing obstacles to a dream these people have and a decision that has already been made.

However, it is important to consider what's holding the patient back from starting. If a patient doesn't want to start treatment because they're going overseas on a family vacation for the next two months, calling them every week before they leave would be annoying. Some people may want to begin treatment for their child when the school year is over. In these cases, it is important to make good notes in their file and set reminders to connect with them when the timing is right.

## What's the Best Way to Follow Up?

For your TC to track and follow up with pending patients efficiently, you must have a system in place to ensure that it's consistent and patients don't get lost. They will need to be able to generate an up-to-date list of the pending patients, their contact information, and any notes that describe their objections to starting treatment.

The majority of offices I've worked with have their TCs tracking their pending patients in an excel spreadsheet. This has been the standard practice in the industry and it works pretty well. There are newer systems that make things easier and more efficient for the whole team, but before we get into that, let's talk about how to use an excel spreadsheet to keep on top of your pendings.

Kasey, Vanessa, and Mary—the wonderful TCs who volunteered to contribute to this book—all use excel spreadsheets to track and follow up with pending patients.

Kasey from Fishbein says:

> "Every single new patient in the Patient Care Center is tracked in an excel spreadsheet. So if a new patient did the exam but doesn't want to start today, the TC makes notes to go back to that Excel sheet to keep track of them, and it's easier to call that way. Also, this is how we determine bonuses for our TCs: we see how many pending patients started within that month by looking at their spreadsheet, and they are rewarded accordingly."

Mary from AllSmiles explains:

> "We have an Excel spreadsheet named "Pending" where we put all the patients who haven't started. We call this our tracker. Each TC gets their own tracker, and they must ensure that they add each pending patient to the list and follow up with them until they give you a firm 'yes' or 'no' answer. It works for us pretty well."

And Vanessa from Knecht reveals:

> "I use an excel spreadsheet to track all my patients: scheduled patients, patients who have decided to start, and patients who haven't started. It's all color-coordinated since it's for my eyes only to keep track of it. For patients that have had their consultations but haven't started, I'll highlight them in bright yellow. That way, I can see it every day, and I can always keep track of who to follow up with regularly until I get them to say 'yes' to a start. And it'll be either a phone call checking in asking if they have questions or a quick text message letting them know we're there for them when they're ready to start treatment."

As you can see, they all have their own methods and reasons for keeping the excel spreadsheet for tracking and following up with patients. Here's the thing with the excel spreadsheet:

it's organized and efficient, but it is not automated and it requires a lot of manual steps. What I mean is, when your TC makes changes in their own spreadsheet, like adding notes after a call, who started, who is still pending, and who declined, it doesn't automatically sort by day or month. It doesn't automatically push out text messages to nurture the lead into a new patient. It doesn't create tasks for follow-up or show you any type of reporting metrics that would show your entire team's activities and conversions. The TC has to take time out of their day to constantly update its information, and they have to keep adding the new pending patients to the list.

Now let's talk about how a system that actively tracks pending patient interactions can make follow-up easier for the whole office.

## Remember PracticeBeacon?

If you've read Front Desk Secrets, you have already been introduced to our CRM System, PracticeBeacon (PB). If your scheduling coordinators are already using it, your TC may already be familiar with what it is and what it does. PB is mostly used by scheduling coordinators for tracking and following up with leads they are trying to schedule for new patient consultations. We've developed a new system so TCs can also use it for tracking and following up with pending patients. Their information is already in the system and it is simply a matter of moving the new patients through a workflow so that scheduling coordinators, treatment coordinators, the operations manager—or anyone who is involved in patient care—can see that patient's status at a glance.

## Here's What the Workflow Looks Like

The scheduling coordinator uses PB to contact prospective patients from the "Leads" column. If the patient agrees to schedule a consultation, the scheduling coordinator moves them to the "Appointment Scheduled" column, and the TC takes over. The TC takes that new patient and goes through the consultation. The new patient either agrees, declines, or waits to start treatment. If they agree, the TC moves the patient to the "Started Treatment" column.

## Getting Started with PB for Pending Patients

If you've been using PB in conjunction with the Excel spreadsheet, all the leads that have booked consultations since you started using PB have probably ended up in the "Appointment Scheduled" column. Why would anyone bother moving them any further? You may have several hundred or more names in that column being a mix of people who should be sorted into "Started Care," "Declined Care," "Observation," and "Pending." Your team will need to do a clean up on the "Appointment Scheduled" column before the system is ready to go.

Once your team is used to sorting the new patient consultations into the approprate columns, your TC can check the "Pending" column daily to see who they need to follow up with today. What's so great about PB is that you can phone or text a patient right from the system and all contacts are recorded by the software. The notes section can be viewed by anyone on your team and everyone knows what is happening with each patient.

## If Your TC Insists on Working from a Spreadsheet

Your TC can easily export the most recent data to an Excel Spreadsheet and use it to make their calls and build reports. If some of the patients are from referrals or Google searches and did not get added to PB by the scheduling coordinator, they should be added to PB so all patient information is consolidated in one system.

Here are a few advantages when using PB to track and follow up with pending patients:

- The entire team is using the same system.
- Everything is in one place, centralizing all the data.
- It's constantly updated and active.
- You can phone, email, or text directly from PB.
- Everyone can see where the patient is in the pipeline.
- You get an accurate picture of your practice growth at a glance.
- It's insanely easy.

Using PB for tracking and following up is the next level of training we're giving our practices. You just heard it here first!

## Keep in Touch!

If your TC is feeling down about not making the sale right away, I encourage you to remind them of this: Pending patients want to start treatment, otherwise they would never have scheduled the exam. If they're following up with pending patients once a week for at least a month, the odds of conversion are still good.

Did you know that only 44% of the leads we generate for our patients will ever be called or followed up on more than once? Yet, 93% of conversions happen after the 6th touchpoint. Math aside, this basically means that the more your team follows up with pending patients, the more likely they will be sitting in your chair. Make sure your TC is following up consistently via phone or text message. A simple call or message is really all that is needed to let the patient know you're thinking about them and looking forward to seeing them when they're ready.

## Reactivation Campaigns

We already know that fees are the biggest obstacle preventing new patients from starting treatment. One way to overcome this is to have your TC reach out to pending patients to tell them about promotions and incentives going on that month! We call this a reactivation campaign. Are you planning on doing a down payment match for June? Let them know! Did you receive a new stock of Gobi toothbrushes this week? Text or call them about the give-away you have for all new starts while supplies last!

The easiest way to do this is by using PB. If your team is using it to schedule new leads and plans to use it to track and follow up with pending and existing patients, PB really is your secret weapon for practice success. It's so simple. Just go to all the columns in PB where patients aren't currently scheduled to start, such as "Pending" or "Recall," "Interested," "No-Show," or even "Declined Treatment" (because why not take your shot again?). They are added to the automated reactivation campaign and get dripped texts and emails about promotions happening in your office. By training your scheduling team to respond immediately to those who answer, you can get those people back on your schedule.

Here's an example of a reactivation campaign text message via PB:

- *Hey there, (prospective patient's name)! Still interested in orthodontic treatment? There's no better time than now to get started! This week only, (practice's name) is offering $1250 off braces or Invisalign! This offer won't last, so reply "YES" now and a member of our team will reach out to schedule your appointment.*

Vanessa from Knecht knows how effective reactivation campaigns can be to get patients back on board:

*"If I haven't heard from a patient in a while, I'll send them a promotional offer via PracticeBeacon. The last time I did it, it was about $500 off. They called me as soon as they received it in their email, and we got them started the following day. People are busy, and sometimes they forget. Or they're just so concerned about the money, and they're waiting for you to budge a bit. The reactivation campaigns are super successful, so I always take advantage of it with my pending patients if there's a promotion going on. Works like a charm every time."*

Take it from Dr. Farina himself from Farina Orthodontic Specialists. He recently partnered with HIP and scheduled 65-70 prospective patients and started 50 from one single reactivation campaign. To hear his story and learn more about reactivation campaigns, scan this QR code.

## Just Make Sure the Follow-Up Gets Done

No matter what system you decide to go with, make sure the follow-up happens consistently. It works like magic and puts money in the bank. All it takes is having the proper systems in place. We're excited to work with our current practices on transitioning to PB for all their patient tracking and follow up needs. We think it is the best way to keep everything streamlined and efficient for the ultimate growth of your practice!

If you're feeling just a little overwhelmed by all the different processes and scripts involved in staying on top of leads, new patients, and pending starts, don't worry. In the next chapter, we've pulled it all together for you. You'll see how the scheduling coordinator, TC, and orthodontist work together to take an online lead all the way through to starting treatment.

CHAPTER **7**

# Tying It All Together

*"You don't have to be great to start, but you have to start to be great."*

*– Zig Zigler*

By this point in The Orthodontic Practice Growth Series, you've learned what your front desk and scheduling coordinators should do to efficiently get leads booked for their new patient consultation. You've also learned what your TC should do to eliminate your patient's fears and objections to get more same-day starts.

I know, there are a lot of strategies and concepts to remember and you and your team are very busy. For the sake of time, I thought it would be best to pull all the strategies together from Books 1 and 2 so you have a place to reference the whole process, start to finish, of taking a lead from first contact to starting treatment.

Let's introduce the fictional main characters from Smith Orthodontics who will be taking us on this journey:

> Andrea - Online Lead
> Mona - Front Desk Coordinator
> Jan - Scheduling Coordinator
> Sally - Treatment Coordinator
> Carmen - Records Technician
> Dr. Smith - Orthodontist

## Andrea Wants a New Smile

Andrea wants nothing more than to fix her crooked teeth so she can express herself fully with a big smile displaying all her pearly whites. After years of feeling self-conscious about her teeth and avoiding photographs, Andrea is ready to make a change and feel confident with her smile. She begins her Google search looking for orthodontic practices in her area. *So many options*, she thinks to herself. So, she looks for the one whose website looks the most professional and has the best customer reviews. Andrea stumbles upon Smith Orthodontics in her search and comes across dozens of positive Google reviews:

> *"I have had the best experience at Smith Orthodontics over these last two years. The team really made me feel comfortable and confident in my decision to get treatment. I'm so happy with my results and I couldn't thank Dr. Smith and his wonderful team enough. I couldn't recommend their practice more!"*

> *"Thank you, Jan, Sally, Dr. Smith, and everyone else who helped me along the way during my treatment. You guys are rockstars!! I'm recommending everyone I know."*

> *"If you need braces or Invisalign, go see Dr. Smith and his team. They changed my life."*

*Okay, looks promising.* Andrea clicks their website link and the first thing she notices is that treatment starts as low as $300 down payment and $149/month. This stood out to her as she's been curious about the cost of treatment, but the other websites didn't provide any indication as to how much it would be. *That's not bad, I think I can make that work.* She browses through the site some more and comes across the "Request a Free Consultation" tab. She enters in her information and receives the message, "Our scheduling coordinator will be in touch with you shortly!" Two minutes later, her phone rings.

80

**Andrea:** Hello?

**Jan:** Hi, is this Andrea?

**Andrea:** Yes, speaking.

**Jan:** Hi! This is Jan from Smith Orthodontics.

**Andrea:** Oh, hi! That was so fast.

**Jan:** We're quick here! How are you today?

**Andrea:** I'm good, thanks. How are you?

**Jan:** I'm doing well, thanks for asking. I see you requested a free consultation at our office? Is that right?

**Andrea:** Yes, I've been thinking about fixing my teeth for a while so I thought I would start looking into it.

**Jan:** Great to hear! I can help you start that process! Is this a good time to talk?

**Andrea:** Yes, for sure.

Jan briefly fills Andrea in about Dr. Smith and their philosophy towards optimal patient care and treatment. She asks her some rapport-building questions to determine how she found their practice, and gathers all of the required new patient information to put in the system. After a few minutes of discussion, Andrea is curious to know more about the pricing structure that she saw on their website:

**Andrea:** *I noticed on your website that you offer payment plans for treatment. I can't remember what it said exactly, but is that right? And is that just for braces, or Invisalign, as well?*

**Jan:** *Yes, we offer payment plans for all of our treatments. We have to see you to provide a treatment plan with accurate fees, but treatment typically starts at $300 down and $149/month. Would something like that work for you?*

**Andrea:** *Oh, great to hear. Yes, it would.*

**Jan:** *Great. So, now that I have all your info, let's talk a bit about the free consultation.*

Jan proceeds to tell Andrea everything she should expect from the consultation:

> **Jan:** *When you come in, you will meet with our awesome Treatment Coordinator, Sally. You'll take some photos and x-rays, and the doctor will review the findings and make some treatment recommendations. The consultation is free of charge to you. Please allow an hour for your appointment. If Dr. Smith does think that you're ready for treatment, we can actually go ahead and get your treatment started that same day so that you do not have to come back for another appointment, if that is convenient for you?*
>
> **Andrea:** *Great! That sounds awesome. It really is convenient because it's hard to get time off work during the day.*
>
> **Jan:** *Yes, that is the feedback I'm getting from most patients. We're happy to provide the same-day start option! We can see you for your consultation as early as tomorrow. Does the morning or afternoon work for you?*
>
> **Andrea:** *The morning is better, but tomorrow won't work. Do you have anything available the following day?*
>
> **Jan:** *Yes, of course! How about 9:00 am?*
>
> **Andrea:** *That works for me.*
>
> **Jan:** *Great! I'm going to email you the documents and forms you'll need to fill out and send back to us. It should only take around 10 minutes to complete. If you can do that prior to your appointment, that would be perfect.*
>
> **Andrea:** *Sure, not a problem.*
>
> **Jan:** *Perfect. We will see you this Friday at 9:00 am for your free consultation. I'll send you a reminder an hour before your appointment.*
>
> **Andrea:** *Thank you, Jan. It was nice speaking with you.*
>
> **Jan:** *You, as well! Have a great day.*

Andrea wakes up the morning of her consultation to a text message from Smith Orthodontics:

*Hey, Andrea! We are looking forward to seeing you at 9:00 am today! If you need directions, here is a link to our listing. This should open on maps and bring you straight to us! Let me know if you have any questions.*

*P.S. Ask for Jan when you get here!*

*These people are on the ball,* she thinks to herself. Andrea gets ready for her consultation and makes her way to Smith Orthodontics.

## Jan: The Rockstar Scheduling Coordinator

You may have noticed a few strategies Jan implements in her conversation with Andrea:

- She chunked information down to make things more digestible for her.
- She only asked the questions she needed for the initial phone call and directly answered Andrea's questions without diluting them with unnecessary information.
- She carried the conversation with a friendly and upbeat tone, while maintaining a bit of skeptical optimism (E.g., "I see you requested a free consultation. Is that right?").
- She sent her the forms prior to the appointment to save time during the consultation.

You may have also noticed Jan following the "Speed to Lead" strategy:

- She contacted her two minutes after she made her consultation request on the website (the benchmark is five minutes).
- She got her scheduled for her new patient consultation within 48 hours (the benchmark is 72 hours).

Since Andrea answered right away, Jan didn't have to call frequently or leave multiple voicemails. If she didn't answer, the best practice for Jan would have been to touch base with Andrea at least 6 times until she heard a response. Also, Andrea was able to come in for the consultation within the desired time frame, but if she wasn't able to, Jan could have offered a virtual consultation to make the process more convenient for her. In this case, Jan was quite thorough and easily accommodated Andrea, so the process was quite simple. Go Jan!

## Andrea Arrives for Her Free Consultation

Bright and early for the first appointment of the day, Andrea arrives at Smith Orthodontics for her free consultation. When she walks through the doors, she is warmly greeted by Mona at the front desk who helps Andrea with the check-in process. Just as she's about to ask for Jan, two women appear walking down the hallway towards Andrea. One of them calls out, "Andrea! Hi, I'm Jan! We spoke on the phone. It's nice to meet you! How are you doing this morning? "I'm great, thanks. How are you?," Andrea responds. "I'm doing great! This is Sally," she says, gesturing to the woman beside her, "Our amazing Treatment Coordinator. She's going to be running the consultation today. You'll be in good hands." As Andrea and Sally greet each other, another woman approaches. Sally steps in, "And this is the lovely Carmen! She's going to be taking your records today. You'll actually start with her, okay? And when you're done, I'll meet you in the consultation room and we'll go through the process." "Okay, great. Thank you." Carmen guides Andrea to the consultation room. "Just come in here and we'll get started!"

Since Jan is the amazing scheduling coordinator that she is, she made sure to ask Andrea for her dentist's office number in the documents she had to fill out prior to the appointment.

Yesterday, Jan got in touch with her dentist's receptionist and got her to send Andrea's most recent x-rays, which were only taken a few months ago. Jan quickly forwarded the x-ray images to Carmen and the doctor already had a good look at them. So, lucky for Carmen, she only has to take photos of Andrea's teeth today, cutting the time in half. The records portion of the exam only ended up taking 4 minutes instead of the targeted 8 minutes. Great teamwork, right? Carmen sends the photos to the doctor for review and invites Sally back to the room. "Sit tight, Sally will be back shortly with the doctor."

## What If the Patient Doesn't Have Up-to-Date X-Rays?

If Jan wasn't able to retrieve the x-ray results or they didn't exist, the next part of the process would be to take x-rays of Andrea's teeth. However, this shouldn't take more than 3-4 minutes if done properly. So, make sure your record technicians are only taking the necessary x-rays required and practice setting up the machines quickly so it's not taking up too much of the exam time. You can have them practice this with other people on your team, time them, and even reward them when they reach the goal time!

## Andrea Meets Dr. Smith

Sally walks into the room with Dr. Smith. He has viewed the x-rays provided by her dentist and observed the photos sent by Carmen a few minutes prior.

> **Sally:** *Hey, Andrea. This is Dr. Smith. He's going to go over the results and recommend your treatment options.*
>
> **Dr. Smith:** *Hi, Andrea. It's nice to meet you. How are you doing today?*
>
> **Andrea:** *So far so good, thank you!*
>
> **Dr. Smith:** *Great. I've reviewed your records and there are two*

*options we can offer you. If you were interested in braces, you would be in treatment for 24 months and you would have to come in every 6 weeks to get your wires adjusted until the end of treatment. If you were interested in Invisalign, it would be the same length of time but your treatment would look a bit different. It would require you to wear aligners 24 hours a day, but you can take them out when you eat or brush. You will be provided with a set of aligners—all are different and are meant to be worn in specific order. We will let you know when to change aligners. If, by the end of treatment, a couple of teeth still need adjustments, we will provide you with a few more refinement trays.*

Andrea: *Okay, I'm more interested in Invisalign. I'm a little worried about wearing metal braces at 33 years old! *laughing**

**Dr. Smith:** *chuckling* Well, we do have many adults wearing metal braces, so you wouldn't be alone! But we have both options available to you, so it's whatever you prefer. I'll let Sally take it from here to discuss the details and fees. It was nice to meet you and I hope to work with you soon!*

**Andrea:** *Thanks, Dr. Smith. Take care!*

*Dr. Smith leaves the room*

## Doctors! Get In and Get Out, or... Don't Come at All?

As you can see above, Dr. Smith didn't stay very long. He introduced himself and went directly into treatment options. He didn't give a long description of what was wrong with Andrea's smile. She knows she wants to improve her smile, and he's showing her what he can do to fix it. That's it. He politely exits, transitioning the conversation back to Sally. Or, if you recall from earlier, there's the option of going completely doctorless by doing a TC Empowerment Consultation. It seems like Dr. Smith is pretty good at keeping things short and sweet, or maybe he didn't know this was even an option. But several offices I know are already doing this, like Fishbein Orthodontics. Here's what Madison from Fishbein had to say about it:

*"Because I started off at Fishbein as a Clinical Assistant and eventually became a Treatment Coordinator, I had a lot of clinical knowledge. When we decided to implement the TC Empowerment Consultation, where all the TCs now provide the treatment plan to the patient without the doctor being there, I thought I had a huge advantage since I'm already pretty good at explaining the different types of treatments. Our TCs are all learning more of that now so they can feel confident sharing it with the patient. The doctor will tell us the treatment plan, and then we have to go back and explain it to the patient. It saves the doctor a lot of time because they can just continue to provide treatment to the patients in the chair, without getting interrupted by consultations that we are totally capable of handling ourselves. It comes down to confidence and feeling equipped enough to do it, which we all are over here."*

Additionally, Madison also told us how going doctorless has actually helped their conversion rates:

*"The conversion rate actually has gone up since we've gone doctorless. Doctors are just very technical. So whenever our doctors would come in, we would have to constantly remind them that they only have two minutes with the patient. But sometimes, they just start getting too technical, saying things like, "We're gonna rotate this tooth this many degrees," or "We're going to do this many millimeters of expansion." The more information the doctor was giving to the patient, or the parent of the patient, the more overwhelming it became for them. So I think it was a little bit intimidating for the patients to have the doctor in there. So, conversion rates have gone up and consultation times have gone down. And the best part is that our patient's have not been pushing back on this. We've maybe had like two or three patients who have asked for the doctor, which is no big deal—we'll just go grab the doctor. So it's been pretty seamless and quite the benefit, for sure."*

Okay, let's get back to our scenario. It's Sally's time to shine!

## Sally Outlines the Four Commitments to Andrea

In order for a person to commit to a lengthy process involving a large sum of money, the following four factors must be part of their decision-making process. Let's recall what these are:

1.  Do they have the **time** to follow through with the process and get results?
2.  Do they have an **understanding** of how the process works?
3.  Do they have the **authority** to make the decision?
4.  Do they have the **money** to pay for it?

Now let's see how Sally does it:

> **Sally:** *Okay, Andrea, so you're interested in the Invisalign treatment, right?*
>
> **Andrea:** *Yeah, I think that would be the best option for me at this time.*
>
> **Sally:** *Great. Before we get into the pricing, I just want to make sure you're clear on a few things so you understand the commitments you need to make prior to starting Invisalign. Okay?*
>
> **Andrea:** *Sure.*
>
> **Sally:** *Once we begin treatment, you will have to come for check-ups every 8-10 weeks during the 24 months of your treatment for us to analyze your progress. You will also have to come for check-ups for retainer fittings after treatment is over for at least 6 months to a year. Do you think this is something you can commit to?* **[Time]**
>
> **Andrea:** *Yes, that shouldn't be a problem.*
>
> **Sally:** *As the doctor mentioned, you would have to wear the aligners every day for the entire treatment duration, except when eating, drinking anything but water, and brushing, and you would have to change the aligner when directed. It is imperative or else you will not see the results, or you might see them slower than usual. Is this something you think can*

*follow?* **[Understanding]**

**Andrea:** *Absolutely.*

**Sally:** *Great. Jan said that you would be taking care of the treatment cost. Is that still the case, or is there anybody else that might be involved in the financial decision?* **[Authority]**

**Andrea:** *Nope, just me. I will be covering it, but I also have insurance.*

**Sally:** *Perfect, and yes, we've already taken into account your insurance information. Alright, if that all sounds good, this is where we would go over the financial agreement, if that feels appropriate to you?* **[Money]**

**Andrea:** *Sounds good.*

# Sally Presents the Fee Presentation

Now that Andrea has fully understood and committed to the treatment above, Sally can now present the fee presentation. Here's what it looks like: a simple piece of paper with the necessary blanks to fill in Andrea's pertinent information and the treatment fees.

---

Smith Orthodontics Financial Agreement

Date: <u>June 17, 2022</u>          Start Date: <u>June 17, 2022</u>
Responsible Party: <u>Andrea Doe</u>    Phone Number: <u>321-123-2134</u>
Patient: <u>Andrea Doe</u>          Email: <u>adoe@gmail.com</u>
_____ Full Treatment _____ Phase I _____ Phase II _____ ETT
_____ Limited Treatment   x _____ Invisalign _____ Incognito
1. Professional Fee                    $ <u>7000.00</u>
2. Less Applicable Courtesy <u>5</u> %    $ <u>350.00</u>
3. Less Estimated Insurance            $ <u>2500.00</u>
4. Estimated Responsible Party Portion  $ <u>4150.00</u>
5. Less Initial Payment [Due <u>June 17, 2022</u>] $ <u>300.00</u>
6. Unpaid Balance                      $ <u>3850.0</u>

Unpaid balance [#6] above is payable to <u>Smith Orthodontics</u> in <u>24</u> monthly installments of $ <u>160.42</u> each, and one installment of the remaining balance. The first initial payment is payable on <u>July 17, 2022</u> and subsequent installments on the same day of each consecutive month until paid in full. A $10 late fee will be charged on all accounts that are 10 days past due.


<u>Sally Johns</u>        _____        <u>June 17, 2022</u>
Signature            Witness                      Date

---

**Sally:** *Okay, Andrea. Here is your orthodontic financial agreement.*

*Presents this sheet of paper filled out with information*

*This is your total treatment fee.*

*Points to $7000, but doesn't say the number out loud*

*Here's some really good news. We have a promotion going on for the month of June. All new patients get a discount of 5% off their total treatment fee, which is $350. You've got awesome insurance that will cover $2500. That leaves you with $4150. You can take care of that however you want, but just as a starting place to make it easy and convenient for you, if you put down $300 today, your monthly payment will be $160.42/ month over the next 24 months. Is that something that might possibly work for you?*

**Andrea:** *All of that sounds fine. I'm just a little concerned about paying the $300 today. I don't know if I'll be able to dish out that much right now.*

**Sally:** *That's okay... Would you be able to put down $150 today and $150 in two weeks' time?*

**Andrea:** *Yeah if that's possible. At least it'll be after another paycheck.*

**Sally:** *Totally understand, we can easily do that for you.*

*Sally changes #5 on the financial agreement to say $150 due June 17, 2022, and $150 due July 1, 2022*

**Sally:** *Okay, great. And I put the start date on the financial agreement as today's date. Jan mentioned that she told you about our same-day start option and that you were happy to do that. Is that still the case?*

**Andrea:** *Yes, she mentioned it a couple of times. I'm so excited to start treatment today. I'm ready to get the process started!*

**Sally:** *Perfect. Glad to hear! And for getting started today, we're actually going to throw in a Gobi toothbrush as a thank you!*

**Andrea:** *Oh, that's awesome! Thank you.*

**Sally:** *My pleasure. We will call you in two weeks' time to get the payment information for the remaining $150 over the phone. How do you want to take care of the $150 down payment today? Amex or Visa?*

**Andrea:** *Sounds good. Visa is fine.*

**Sally:** *All that's left to do is sign the financial agreement and we'll get started!*

**Andrea:** *Great, I am excited to get started!*

*Andrea signs the agreement*

And that's it, folks. Sally did a fine job presenting all the pricing information in an easy, digestible manner. She gave Andrea the option to split her down payment in half to better accommodate her current financial situation, and she threw in a free gift for starting treatment that same day. It's a pretty straightforward process when you put it all together, right?

## The Treatment Coordinator Checklist

With a bit of guidance and practice, your TC can work just as smoothly and efficiently as Sally in no time. However, we know it's a lot of information to understand and process. It's sometimes difficult to remember the critical steps in the process, so providing your TC with the proper checklist will help them ensure they're doing their role at 100% every time. We want them to be a master of their trade, so we've created a checklist for you. Your TC should be using this daily to ensure that they follow the same process for each potential patient. If they execute this checklist for all new patient requests, you WILL see an increase in new patient starts, guaranteed!

The checklist looks like this:

1. Before patients get to the office, your scheduling coordinators should...

   - Respond to incoming consultation requests in less than 5 minutes.

   - Schedule their in-office consultation within the next 72 hours.

- Offer a virtual exam option to all online consultation requests if they can't be scheduled within 72 hours.
- Pre-frame the fees and same-day start option.

2. At the in-office consult, be sure your TC...

- Limits the doctor's portion of the consult to 5 minutes or less.
- Completes the entire consultation in 30-45 minutes.
- Offer SAME-DAY STARTS to boost conversions.
- Is incentivized with a commission for starts and same-day starts.

3. To overcome price objections, your TC needs to...

- Offer a single, easy-to-understand payment plan.
- Limit your payments to $300 down and $200 monthly (max).
- Offer a high-value incentive for saying YES today.
- Be FLEXIBLE: do whatever it takes to get the YES before they leave.

4. And if your TCs don't get the yes today...

- Don't give up! Follow up with each patient weekly for 1 month.
- Offer attractive incentives to come back and start treatment.

Scan this QR code to view the Treatment Coordinator Checklist PDF so you can print it for your TC!

SCAN ME

There you have it. I have shown you what the nation's top 1% orthodontic practices are doing to get all the new patients they need to hit their production goals. Now it's up to you to apply what you've learned. Once you've implemented the systems I've shared, you'll start growing faster and easier. The next step is for you to decide how big you want to grow.

# CHAPTER 8

# Visualizing Your Future Plans

*"We cannot solve our problems with the same thinking we used when we created them."*

— Albert Einstein

When it comes to growing their practices, most orthodontists immediately jump to their need for new patients. This brings us back to the main subject of Book 1, *Front Desk Secrets*, which was all about training your scheduling coordinator to be a master at responding to leads in 5 minutes or less and getting them booked for a free consultation within 72 hours. This book, *The Ultimate Treatment Coordinator,* was picked up from there to help you groom a TC who can turn those free consultations into starts. With those two key steps in the process under our belt, we can now talk about making headway on your production goals.

When your team has mastered the concepts in the first two books of the Orthodontic Practice Growth Series, then your need for new patients will be handled. Problem solved, right? Now you can grow to the level of production you need to achieve your goal. Well, it's actually not that straightforward. How big you want to grow dictates the business strategy you need to follow to get there.

## What Growth Looks Like Numerically

Over the past eight years, I've had the opportunity to study over a thousand orthodontic practices. At the time of this writing, HIP is actively working with over 140 practices to help them achieve their production goals. As far as size goes, I have broken it down by production numbers which I have defined arbitrarily as small, medium, and large practices. A small practice is defined as anything below three million in production. A medium practice does between three and eight million in production. A large practice is anything over eight million (Disclaimer: this is my criteria not necessarily the industries... but stay with me as I explain why).

| Practice Size | Annual Production |
|:---:|:---:|
| Small | $3,000,000 or less |
| Medium | $3,000,000 to $8,000,000 |
| Large | Over $8,000,000 |

All of these practice sizes are achievable by a solo orthodontist. I've seen it done. However, I do suggest bringing on an associate within the medium size. The question is, how big do you want to grow? What's your number? There's no right or wrong answer here. It really depends on your goals and the lifestyle you want this practice to support.

Next, how are you going to fit all the new patients and follow-up visits into your schedule? Growth causes problems because it disrupts the status quo. Your current systems and procedures support the current volume in your office but they will not work for you at the next level.

> *"In order to take our lives to the next level, we must realize that the same pattern of thinking that has gotten us to where we are now will not get us to where we want to go."*
>
> *– Tony Robbins*

Every level of growth presents a new set of problems that we have to solve with a new mindset. Before we get into the models of different practice sizes, let's just look at the problems that arise when you simply throw more leads at a practice and the logistical solutions that can be used to handle them.

Let's say you've chosen your number and you see that you have some growth to do. You have been stuck at your current volume for a while and have decided the problem is that you don't have enough new patients. Let's call this Problem #1.

You just need more new patients. What is Solution #1? Hire a marketing company to get you leads.

The marketing company is showing you that they are getting results. Your ads are getting clicks to your website and web forms are getting filled out requesting free consultations. We have a new problem. Let's call it Problem #2. Your practice does not seem to be growing despite all the money you're spending on lead generation and you're beginning to wonder about this marketing company. Your staff thinks the leads are low quality and don't seem motivated to follow up with them.

What's Solution #2? Train your front desk on "Speed to Lead" and the concepts in Front Desk Secrets. You follow our recommendations, and your scheduling coordinator is now responding to the leads in five minutes or less and booking them for free consultations within 72 hours.

The next problem arises because your scheduling coordinator is doing a great job of booking the leads from your marketing. Problem #3: We don't have enough room in our schedule for all the free consultations.

We actually had a practice that called us up and fired us after six months of doing their marketing because they were too busy and booked out for months! I was disappointed that we did not get to help them solve the next-level problems with their operations, but I was happy that they seemed to have grasped "Speed to Lead."

Solution #3 is the topic of this book. It's all about getting your TC to be able to do 30-minute consultations and convert them into same-day starts. You get your team on board with the idea and get everyone to specialize in their roles. You diligently apply everything you've learned in the previous chapters and you've doubled your capacity for consultations.

Dr. Kyle Sparkman of Sparkman Orthodontics got referred to HIP because he needed a new website. He's been in practice for 16 years, has 3 doctors, and 3 locations.

Within 2 months they got so busy that they were booked out for 6 weeks and had to ask us to turn advertising off until they could catch up. We worked with them to cut their exam time in half with the 30-minute consultation and we're able to get the advertising back up and running.

I just got a message from him saying they had a record month with 211 starts!

Your practice is growing, the team is motivated, and the morale is good. The thing is, your scheduling coordinator is doing such a great job that all your free consultation slots are booked three weeks out. The next problem, Problem #4, is that a lot of these appointments are no shows. This is understandable with our instant gratification culture. People keep calling around until they find someone who can take them sooner and neglect to give us a courtesy call to tell us they aren't coming. They're not highly invested in showing up since it was a free consultation.

Solution #4, which is also covered in this book, is to offer people a virtual consultation when you can't get them scheduled within the 72-hour window. This screens out the people who aren't serious about starting or can't afford treatment. It also helps the appointments that are booked further out to stick because they already feel involved with your office. It increases the conversion rate because these new patients are pre-screened and of higher quality.

Now you're seeing the growth you want and production is moving upwards towards your goal. The practice is much busier and you have your hands full with all the follow-ups. Problem #5 is that you have a hard time pulling away from chair time to go do consultations.

Solution #5 is the TC Empowerment (Doctorless) Consultation. You train your TC to deliver your recommendations from the patient's x-rays and photos. Your TC gets very good at this and increases their conversion rate. As a result, you have more time to spend on treatment which is good because the number of follow-ups you need to do keeps increasing.

Problem #6 occurs when you start feeling like you're reaching the upper limit of follow-ups that you want to do in a day.

Solution #6 involves the use of technology to find solutions to providing follow-up without the patient needing to occupy your chair or take up your time. Check out tech solutions like Dental-Monitoring.com or Rhinogram.com which allow patients to send you photos of their teeth. This allows you to assess their progress faster, without taking up chair time, and provides them the convenience of a check-up without having to disrupt their day.

Dr. Dressler, the founder of Rhinogram, who is also an orthodontist and client of HIP, said:

> *"I have done over 1200 virtual consults in my own practice. Most, if not all patients, know their teeth are crooked and need straightening. They also know the type of treatment they want, braces, clear aligners, etc. The reason for coming in to see you is to see what their insurance covers and if they can afford the treatment. Being able to answer that question 98% of the time from the patient's home will eliminate unnecessary in-office visits and chair time. It also eliminates endless follow up for people who can not afford your care but are too embarrassed to tell you face-to-face, but gladly tell you behind the texting mask."*

If your practice is growing, you should be running into problems. It's a good thing. The question is, how do you anticipate the problems and solve them so you keep moving towards your goal? Let's look at the operational models that orthodontists can use to build the different practice sizes and run them efficiently.

## The Boutique Practice

When an orthodontist graduates, hangs out their shingle, and opens their doors for business, they usually get what we refer to as a boutique practice. It's a nice little practice that reflects the personality and quirks of the doctor. They hit the ground running and tackle problems as they come. Systems get added on as problems come up and they make it work. A practice like this can typically do about 1.2 million in production but with all the competition out there, and all the debt piling up, it can be a struggle.

## Transitioning from Boutique to Business

If the orthodontist realizes that their training made them a great clinical practitioner but not a particularly good business owner, they can begin the transition from a boutique practice to a fast-growing orthodontic business. This involves the doctor admitting that they don't have the answers and they can't do it all themselves. They seek out help in running the business.

Dr. Fishbein believes that orthodontists are good at one thing—being an orthodontist:

> *"I always say orthodontists are typically good at one thing and that's orthodontics. It's also literally the most profitable thing they can be doing with their time. So when you see an orthodontist trying to manage these different areas, typically, they're not great at it. But even more importantly, if they use that time to see patients, it would be a better use of their time, both functionally and financially."*

You've probably noticed that the training implementation necessary to get the processes in this book up and running takes a lot of time. Making the transition from boutique to business comes with the decision that you should not be the one overseeing the implementation and training. In the org chart for a small practice below, you'll notice that the orthodontist is at the top and below them is the office manager. The orthodontist sets the vision for where the practice will go and then delegates it to the office manager to make it happen.

When Dr. Fishbein realized that he needed to hire an Office Manager to oversee the day-to-day operations instead of him, he knew he should promote one of his fantastic team members first:

*"We've always promoted within. Our current COO, Amanda Floyd, who's the best in the business, started as a clinical assistant and I promoted her to office manager. But I remember telling her, 'Hey, I don't have anything left in the budget to pay you.' But I told her what I wanted to do, how I wanted to grow, and every time we did grow, I would pay her more and more. I just outright told her where I wanted to be in 5 years' time in terms of production, and she agreed to do that with me. After the first 12 months of her working in the role, she told me we hit our 5-year mark. I remember her asking, 'So, what's next?'"*

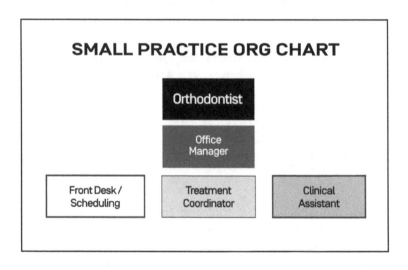

Dr. Kristen Knecht opened the doors to her brand new practice just days before the COVID-19 pandemic hit. She knew Knecht Orthodontics needed a strong brand identity and an enjoyable experience that would convert potential leads into happy patients in her practice from the very beginning. We ensured that her vision for her practice was reflected in her digital platforms using HIP's Brand Identity Process. In addition, Dr. Knecht onboarded the right team members who could truly be brand ambassadors. We then ensured every team member was well versed in our Patient Acquisition and Retention Framework™. Once we were confident they could convert the leads we generated, we launched her marketing campaigns.

Dr. Knecht started her practice with a business mindset from the get-go. She invested heavily into the right people, systems, and marketing upfront, and her investment paid off. In the first ten months after opening her doors during a pandemic, she converted over half a million dollars worth of digital leads into happy patients.

> *"I know doctors who work five or ten years to get to this level, and it's all happened so quickly. I couldn't have done that on my own."*

She produced well over a million dollars in her first full year in practice (2021) and is on pace to produce two million this year. By next year, she will be on track to hire a Chief Operating Officer (COO) and from there, it's up to her how big she wants to grow. It's all a matter of her goals and the lifestyle she wants to live.

Scan this QR code to learn more about Dr. Knecht's case study.

When you look at the medium and large practice org charts, you'll notice that they both involve a COO. Adding this role to your practice is not something that makes financial sense right away. A practice should consider hiring a COO when they reach the three million mark. This is the topic of Book #3 in the Orthodontic Practice Growth Series.

Dr. Fishbein shares his experience and what worked for him as he grew from a boutique practice to his eight locations today:

"It's very easy for me to say that I have a COO, 8 TCs, and a Director of Operations, and all that stuff, because our production and collections are able to justify those needs. But when you're just starting off, and you don't have those collections coming in, you're not going to be able to pay somebody a couple of hundred thousand. I mean, the income's just not there. So when you start off it's not uncommon for you to have a couple team members doing multiple roles. But as you grow, I think it's important that you have those team members in place ready to take on those responsibilities because otherwise you're hindering your growth. So that's why, even in the beginning, I tended to like to be a little bit overstaffed than understaffed, even if that meant cutting my margin a little bit. Because I wasn't so worried about the margin and what I was taking home because I knew that growth was going to help me down the line, which it did."

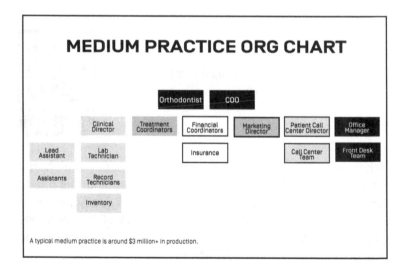

## MEDIUM PRACTICE ORG CHART

Orthodontist — COO

Clinical Director — Treatment Coordinators — Financial Coordinators — Marketing Director — Patient Call Center Director — Office Manager

Lead Assistant — Lab Technician — Insurance — Call Center Team — Front Desk Team

Assistants — Record Technicians

Inventory

A typical medium practice is around $3 million+ in production.

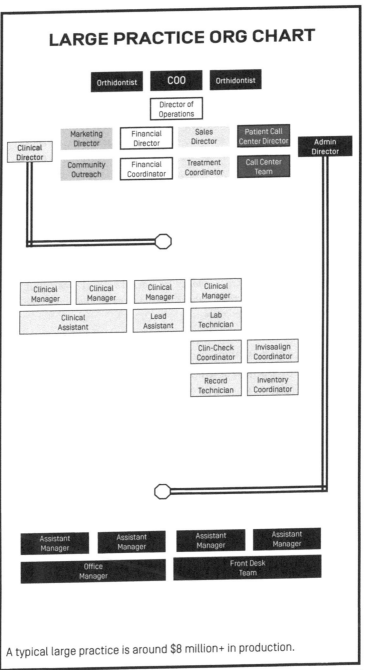

# LARGE PRACTICE ORG CHART

Orthidontist | COO | Orthidontist

Director of Operations

Marketing Director | Financial Director | Sales Director | Patient Call Center Director | Admin Director

Clinical Director

Community Outreach | Financial Coordinator | Treatment Coordinator | Call Center Team

Clinical Manager | Clinical Manager | Clinical Manager | Clinical Manager

Clinical Assistant | Lead Assistant | Lab Technician

Clin-Check Coordinator | Invisaalign Coordinator

Record Technician | Inventory Coordinator

Assistant Manager | Assistant Manager | Assistant Manager | Assistant Manager

Office Manager | Front Desk Team

A typical large practice is around $8 million+ in production.

Dr. Fishbein explains how he was able to grow from a 1 million dollar practice to a 25 million dollar practice in less than ten years:

> "You know, there are so many key performance indicators that people talk about and most of it is just noise to me. Like I hear about 'profit per visit' and 'profit per case' and blah, blah, blah. What we focus on is getting patients in the door and then taking really good care of those patients. And on top of that, taking really good care of our team. So I think if you focus on those things, those very simple things, I think you can grow faster. You can't just focus on all these small key performance indicators and metrics. As the orthodontist, focus on just a few important things and then delegate the other important things to your staff. I think that's one of the things that helped us. There's really no secrets; just keep your patients and your team happy, and delegate tasks to the right people on your team."

If your production is at a level that will support hiring a COO, stay tuned for Book #3 which will be released in the fall of 2022. If you're not quite there yet, that's okay. The strategies in books one and two will have you growing to that level in no time if you and your team are dedicated to getting them up and running. For now, set the vision for how big you want to grow and why, and let's get to work creating the practice and life of your dreams.

# Conclusion

Nothing makes me happier than realizing my mission of living with integrity and helping business owners to make the best decisions with their time, money, marketing, and health. Since 2014, I have had the honor of helping hundreds of orthodontists to build incredible lives by growing their practices and serving their communities.

Serving more people involves so much more than just running more people through your office. It involves showing people that you really care about their wants and needs, wowing them with phenomenal customer service, and making the experience of creating that smile memorable. It starts with your vision and making sure that the practice you are building can deliver on its promise in each and every interaction.

So far in the Orthodontic Practice Growth Series, I've shown you what it takes to fill two critical roles with team members who are dedicated to getting members of your community into your chair to start treatment. Book #1, *Front Desk Secrets*, went in-depth on the scheduling coordinator role, and this book covered everything your TC needs to know to be a master at their role.

If you just need more new patients, marketing for people with crooked teeth is easy. If you want to see those people starting treatment, that takes a little more effort and skill. If you and your team are diligent about implementing what you've learned in this book, you will have no problem getting all the starts you want.

Take the time to train with your team and invite them to grow and celebrate with you. As you get the 5 Growth Hacks up and running in your practice, momentum will build and your team will be excited about breaking records week after week. You'll get to the point where it becomes second nature for them to:

1. Respond to leads in 5 minutes or less and schedule them within 72 hours.
2. Pre-frame fees and same-day starts in the first call.
3. Double capacity with our 30-Minute New Patient Consultation.
4. Get more 'yeses' with our 5-Minute Fee Presentation.
5. Start 80% of new patients the same day with our Proven Playbook.

After that, it's just a matter of how big you want to grow. I've seen the growing pains that the nation's top 1% orthodontic practices have experienced and I've helped them to troubleshoot and grow through them. Whatever size practice you want, there's a successful model for it. Building the practice of your dreams is just a matter of getting out of your own way.

The next logical step in the process is hiring someone whose expertise is in business, leadership, and operations, to run your practice. I hope you'll join me on this journey in Book #3 of The Orthodontic Practice Growth Series which will be released in Fall 2022. It will provide an in-depth look into the best practices for orthodontic operations. If you want to grow your practice to a medium or large scale or if you're looking to remove yourself from management so you can focus on what you do best, make sure to get your hands on a copy.

Until then, enjoy these 5 Growth Hacks and revel in how easy getting new patients really can be!